PLANT SONGS

Reflections on Herbal Medicine

JESSICA BAKER, LAC, RH (AHG)

BALBOA.
PRESS
A DIVISION OF HAY HOUSE

Balboa Press books may be ordered through booksellers or by contacting:

Balboa Press
A Division of Hay House
1663 Liberty Drive
Bloomington, IN 47403
www.balboapress.com
1 (877) 407-4847

Because of the dynamic nature of the Internet, any web addresses or links contained in this book may have changed since publication and may no longer be valid. The views expressed in this work are solely those of the author and do not necessarily reflect the views of the publisher, and the publisher hereby disclaims any responsibility for them.

The author of this book does not dispense medical advice or prescribe the use of any technique as a form of treatment for physical, emotional, or medical problems without the advice of a physician, either directly or indirectly. The intent of the author is only to offer information of a general nature to help you in your quest for emotional and spiritual well-being. In the event you use any of the information in this book for yourself, which is your constitutional right, the author and the publisher assume no responsibility for your actions.

Any people depicted in stock imagery provided by Thinkstock are models, and such images are being used for illustrative purposes only.
Certain stock imagery © Thinkstock.

Print information available on the last page.

ISBN: 978-1-5043-9355-3 (sc)
ISBN: 978-1-5043-9357-7 (hc)
ISBN: 978-1-5043-9356-0 (e)

Library of Congress Control Number: 2017919112

Balboa Press rev. date: 01/26/2018

CONTENTS

PART 4:   ADULTHOOD/WISDOM PLANTS

Dedicated to the Earth, to the Water, to the Mother Vine,
and to every plant and fungus.
I offer these words to you, for all of your nourishment,
inspiration, and wisdom.

INTRODUCTION

As an herbalist, I have had the opportunity to work with herbal medicine for almost twenty years. Most of my early herbal teachers encouraged me to practice the folk method of study. They taught that to "study" a plant is to honor it, sit with it, drink an infusion of some or all of its parts (flower, leaf, bark) and wait for images, messages or sensations to arise. This simple meditation gave me insights into the herbs and into my own psyche. I began to understand that my own feelings of isolation and loneliness were from my lack of connection to nature.

I grew up in a military family, which means we moved at least every two years; sometimes we stayed places only a few months. Lonely doesn't begin to describe what it feels like to always be the "new kid," to have no permanent home, to have no town, city, or state to call my own. When other people spoke of home, my mind conjured no image. When asked where my permanent home was, I always said, "I don't know, I've never had one." The reaction was usually one of pity, with an underlying fear, as people couldn't imagine not having a physical location that embodied "home." My sense of disconnection had a lot to do with not having the ability to set my roots down. I moved to Humboldt County California when I was twenty-one, and among the magnificence of the redwood forests I was guided back home to myself, so that I could finally grow my roots.

As a practitioner, I have also seen loneliness and isolation in many of my clients. When I ask them, "What brings you the most joy?" or, "When do you feel connected or at one with everything?" I hear more often than anything else, "When I am in the forest; on the beach; walking in nature; watching the sunset." It is the act of being in the presence of nature that creates the feeling of connection and inclusion.

I have seen remarkable changes in my clients' health with "simple" instructions such as, "Allow yourself permission to walk on the beach or in the forest for ten minutes a day." For some people, ten minutes of being in nature begins as a chore, because they think of all the things they should be doing. Within weeks this chore becomes an integral part of their days, where they can let go of stress and hassles, breathe in the beauty of their environments, and reflect on what they value out of life. It is often the simplest exercises that have the most profound results.

In my work with clients with PTSD I have found herbalism to play a significant role in healing. As soon as they walk into my clinic the plants start working on them. Essential oils, diffused for their aromatic and disease-fighting properties, hang in the air. The smells of herbs in their jars draw people in. Once my clients are in the treatment room, I may burn incense or perform moxibustion. This revives the lost connection to our plant kin and awakens dormant parts of our beings.

My clients' understanding of their spirits begin to change as they work with the plants, whether it is from growing their own lavender or decocting a medicinal tea. One client was in her early forties when she walked into my community acupuncture clinic. Once I saw her I knew she was in shock and had severe PTSD. As she began to tell her story of being kidnapped and finding what she believed to be her birth family—later she would find out that those parents were also part of the kidnapping—I could see that a lifetime of neglect, abuse, and trauma is not what broke her. She had already spent years working on that. It was the realization that she didn't know who she was that pushed her over the edge. The truth of her kidnapping was recent news and she was not able to assimilate it. Her eyes reflected how lost she was. Her story was so outrageous that she feared I wouldn't believe her.

I did believe her, and for that first treatment I gave her the NADA (National Acupuncture Detox Association) protocol—five auricular points for PTSD, stress, addiction, and withdrawal. She was noticeably more relaxed afterwards. She came back for private or community acupuncture weekly. After the first couple of treatments I gave her a simple herbal formula to strengthen digestion and nourish blood so she could "stomach" the news and support her spirit as she discovered who she really was. After she had been on the formula for a couple of weeks I could tell that the herbs had begun to work. Although she was still traumatized, there were more moments of clarity, acceptance and hope. She discovered many more truths about her identity, her birth family, and the insidious nature of child kidnapping rings, and each time the herbs were there to help her process them.

It is true that her willpower, courage, and spirit ultimately healed her. The acupuncture and my belief in her ability to heal helped. Her already-healthy lifestyle choices also perpetuated her healing. I do believe that without herbal medicine, she may not have progressed as quickly. The subtle fragrance of aromatic plants in my office and her treatments created a safe, healing space. The herbs she ingested allowed her to assimilate nutrients and emotions and also to calm her mind and spirit. The medicine of the plants reminded her that she is loved, nourished and blessed. It took many months of acupuncture and herbs to move her out of the acute phase of trauma as she unraveled the layers of neglect, abuse and fear. Years later I am happy to report that although she still has some days where she experiences some anxiety or sadness, she is thriving. She is healthy, peaceful, and has begun to travel the world.

Nature heals. I have been healed by trees, herbs, and by the sea. The Earth has always provided and will continue to do so if we just listen. Plants have always transformed us. They have kept us alive, evolved cultures, and bound us to other people and places. Most importantly, they are part of us. All living organisms share the same DNA. Our genetic code is more like that of plants than different. We share approximately 60% of our DNA with a banana plant, for example. We are of the same essence, the same source, the same miracle.

Plant Songs is structured so that it can be read as a narrative, moving through the phases of my life, beginning with childhood—Part I: Life Lines—and ending with the present—Part IV: Wisdom Plants. You can also just read one chapter at a time, in any order. I have also included a basic introduction to Chinese medicine theory, a table with a few of the five element correspondences, and definitions for words commonly used in classical Chinese medicine. This will serve as a reference as you read through each chapter.

My motivation and inspiration for *Plant Songs* are the plants themselves. Their messages have come as gifts of remembrance and love, not only for their own sake, but also for ours. The plants know humanity is sick. Their longevity on this Earth vastly surpasses ours and they have seen the extermination and evolution of countless species. They see that humans are reaching a tipping point and they want to help us heal from our societal sickness.

Plants miss the deep connection that humans once had with them. They know our mental and physical illnesses are due to that loss of relationship. They want to remind us that they are here; they are here to help us be nourished, healed, and joyful. My hope is to inspire readers to regain their own connection to plants and our planet. I hope you will remember the divine beauty of each of our plants, as well as your own.

Classical Chinese Medicine: Foundations

Daoists and naturalists believe that when a person lives simply and in cohesion with the cycles of the seasons, the phases of the moon, and the temperaments of the weather, he/she can live an ageless life, peaceful and healthy. They recognize and honor that the rhythms of the Cosmos and the Earth are the same as those within Humanity. Humans are a conduit between Heaven and Earth; our energy—and the energy of all living beings—takes part in the delicate balance of life. When you harmonize with all the cosmic and earthly forces that also embody you, you are in union with the *Dao*. In consonance with the *Dao*, you enter the *Wu Ji* (ultimate void) and from that timeless space you access the infinite energy of the universe.

It is our disconnection from the rhythms of the universe that has caused so much illness and destruction in the world. Before 1,000 BC, most *Wu Xi*, or shaman doctors, were women. The character for *Wu* denotes "above," or "Heaven," and "below," or "Earth." They were the keepers of balance between what is above and what is below. They were called to heal, interpret dreams, spirit travel, perform exorcisms, pray for rain, and in times of disaster, plea to the celestial spirits with chants and wails. The *I-Ching* was the theoretical text for *Qigong* (the cultivation of energy through movement, breath and meditation) training. There was no separation between the study of medicine and divination.

The Zhou Dynasty (1028-221 BC) saw many changes in politics and society. The fertile soil and widespread adoption of agriculture and livestock breeding allowed for abundance. This was a time of intellectual and artistic awakening that in part contributed to a forgetting the ways of the *Dao*. This period was the first time China began to organize clinical medicine into different divisions or departments. The character *Wu* (shaman) was replaced with *Yi* (doctor of medicine). Later, the bottom ideogram was substituted and represented a bottle of wine, for the medical application of herbs. Chinese medicine has become more refined and sophisticated over the last two thousand years, but it is the Daoist roots that hold the essence of how to truly heal. The Daoists' understanding of herbal medicine comes from the intimate connection they had with the plants and all of the natural forces of the universe.

Classical Chinese Medicine: Theory

Five elements/phases: The five elements are deeply engrained in Chinese medicine. They represent the fundamental elements of all natural phenomenon within the universe, including humanity. Each element has correspondences, such as a season, color, musical note, grain, and more. For humans, these include a yin and yang organ, emotion, sound of voice, and spiritual influence.

Element	Season	Organs	Color	Voice	Emotion	Spirit influence
Wood	Spring	Liver Gallbladder	Green	Loud or Shouting	Compassion Anger/Frustration	Hun - ethereal soul
Fire	Summer	Heart/Pericardium Small Intestine/ San Jiao	Red or Pink	Laughing	Joy/Passion Mania	Shen - mind, consciousness
Earth	Late Summer or 18-day shift	Spleen Stomach	Golden Yellow	Singing	Contentment Worry Pensive	Yi - thought, inclination
Metal	Autumn	Lung Large Intestine	White	Crying	Acceptance Grief/Sorrow	Po - corporeal soul
Water	Winter	Kidneys Bladder	Black Dark Blue	Groaning	Courage/Will Fear/Shock	Zhi - will, determination

Yin yang means many things in Chinese medicine. The character for yin is the shady side of the mountain, while yang is the sunny side of the mountain. They are opposites that create wholeness. Yin yang represents an expression of duality of balance and harmony within the body as well as the universe. Yin and yang are dependent on one another, thus all things have a yin and yang aspect to their nature. The balance of yin yang is constantly in flux. This dynamic opposition is responsible for the transformation of the body's vital life-force energy.

Yin	Yang
Night	Day
Earth	Heavens
Moon	Sun
Dense	Light
Material	Immaterial
Wet	Dry
Cold	Hot
Passive	Active
Receptive	Creative
Grows	Generates
Contraction	Expansion

Qi (pronounced "chi") is the vital life force energy that is present in all things. Qi can manifest in various degrees of density, as is represented in the character for Qi, a depiction of steam coming off a cooking pot of rice, as well as the rice itself. Qi can be understood as the different forms of water: vapor, liquid, ice. The strength and motility of our Qi reflects the vitality of our health. There are too many types of Qi to mention, but I will define three:

- **Wei Qi** is the external defensive energy that allows a person to defend from external influences like colds, flus, and allergens.
- **Ying Qi** is the nutritive energy that lies deeper within the body and is affected by how well a person is nourished and cared for.
- **Yuan Qi** is the constitutional energy a person births into this life with and is the foundation of all yin and yang in the body.

Meridians are a series of energetic channels that run throughout the body. They supply Qi to every part of the body, assist in the distribution of blood and body fluids, maintain the balance of yin and yang, and protect against disease. Points along these channels are used to regulate, sedate, or strengthen Qi to achieve balance and health.

Chinese medicine identifies patterns that arise when the body and spirit are out of balance with cosmic and earthly forces. Diagnosis is not the same as in allopathic medicine and emphasis is put on interpreting patterns by looking at the tongue and feeling radial pulses. To describe patterns observed in the body, some of organ names are used to describe them. It is important to remember that when there is a diagnosis of liver qi stagnation that organ names pertain to energetic layers in the body, not only the physical organ.

PART I

Early Childhood/Life Lines

Magnolia, Pine, Oak, and Rose

Growing up in a military family meant moving every time my dad was "stationed" somewhere else. Stationary is not the word that describes the feeling of being uprooted as soon as you begin to feel comfortable where you are. By the time I was seven or eight, a sense of loneliness began to settle in me. I began to see people and places as temporary and impermanent, and that shaped the relationship I had with everything, including myself.

The plants I chose in Part I are some of the first plants I began to recognize as familiar presences in my life. I chose Magnolia for the love of my grandmother and Pine for my great-grandfather's land. Oak helps me find strength within myself, and Rose is a reminder of the beauty and love that surrounds me, regardless of where I am.

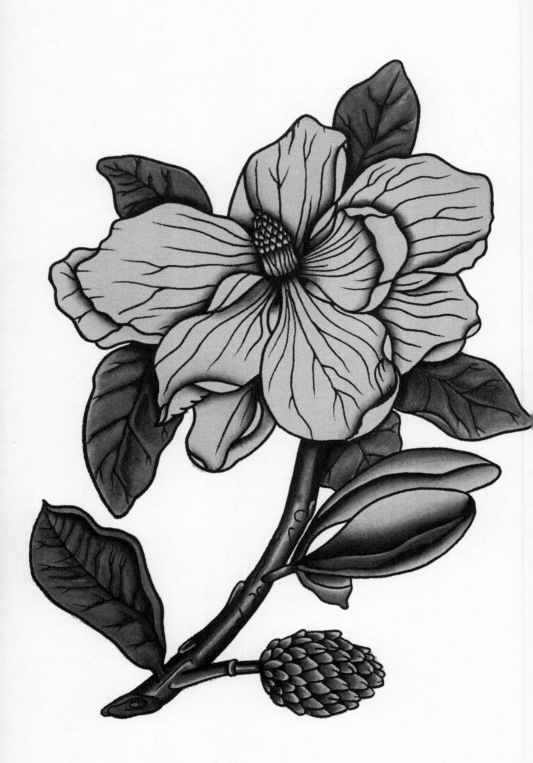

CHAPTER ONE

Magnolia: Breathe Life In

Magnolia liliflora (quinquepeta)
Lily Magnolia
Mu Lan

> **Properties:** Bitter, Cold
> **Meridians entered:** Large Intestine, Lung, Spleen, Stomach
> **Original habitat:** Fujian, Hubei, Sichuan and NW Yunnan provinces
> **Habitats:** Slopes and forest edges at elevations of 300-1600 meters.

Magnolia officinalis
Magnolia bark
Hou Po

> **Properties:** Bitter, Acrid, Warm, Aromatic
> **Meridians entered:** Large Intestine, Lung, Spleen, Stomach
> **Elements influenced:** Metal, Earth
> **Original habitat:** East Asia; west China
> **Habitats:** Alpine and hilly areas; forests at elevations of 300-1500 meters.

Jessica Baker, LAc, RH (AHG)

Magnolia grandiflora
Southern Magnolia

Properties: Bitter, Aromatic

Meridians entered: Lung, Large Intestine, Spleen

Elements influenced: Metal, Earth

Original habitat: SE North America from North Carolina to Florida to Texas.

Habitats: Hammocks, sand dunes, buffs and sandy bottoms. Rich moist soils at elevations under 105 meters.

Description: Magnolias grow with a pyramidal to rounded cone and can be 60-80 feet tall. They have an evergreen broadleaf with dark green ovate to elliptic leaves. Magnolias have stunning large fragrant flowers that are white, yellow, pink, or purple. The flowers have three sepals and six to twelve flowers in spiral arrangements that flower in the late spring. The fruits are large red and cone-like. Magnolias can live to be up to 120 years old.

> *Breathe life in*
> *Breathe life out*
> *Transform hate into love*
> *Fear into courage*
> *Despair into growth*

Ancestral Medicine

The centerpiece of my grandparents' yard is a magnificent *Magnolia grandiflora*, called the southern magnolia because it saturates the South with its impermeable aroma in the hot, sticky heat of summer. The billowy white flowers, heavy with nectar, entice bees and people to gather close and inhale their sweetness. My maternal grandparents' house was a gathering place for my great-grandmother and her sisters and brothers—my aunts, uncles and cousins who are too numerous to count. During our summer visits to their house my parents, sister and I would pull up in the neighborhood and my excitement would rise. As we neared their driveway I could see the one-story cedar house, which was set back from the road, the display of old people on the front porch, my cousins playing around flowers of all colors, and the brilliant magnolia towering above them all.

As a young child I loved going there because it meant I got to be with my cousins and grandparents. By the time I was a freshman in high school, though, I had lived in five different states as well as a military base outside of Kaiserslautern, Germany, my dad's last station before his retirement from the US Army. After his retirement we headed for Trenton, Georgia, a small conservative town in the northwest corner of the state, nestled in between Sand and Lookout Mountains, with Alabama and Tennessee only a few minutes away to the west and north. After living in Germany it was almost unbearable to be in a small southern town. But I loved living near my family, especially my grandmother.

My grandma Frances was a resilient woman and even in death is the matriarch of our large family. The only child of my great-grandmother Irene Brewer, she grew up close to her large extended family. In the late 1950s and 60s she was a young woman and divorced with three children. By the time I was born in 1976 she had married Thomas Smartt and had another daughter, and the three of them were living in the cedar house with the magnolia tree out front.

My grandfather took great pride in his yard, and in the roses and flowers he tended as an act of love for my grandma. The planting of the magnolia tree was part of that devotion, though more than once I remember her threatening to chop the tree down. Ants and bees hovered around the tree, making it virtually impossible for us kids not to get bitten or stung. One time when I was stung on the foot, she said, "That's it, that tree is coming down!" Thankfully my granddad wouldn't do it. And the magnolia still stands tall.

For me, the tree embodies her. Like the magnolia whose large, striking, white flowers are supported by its shiny tough oblong leaves, my grandmother was attractive and welcoming with an inner strength that sustained us all.

My fondest summertime childhood memories are tagging along with her on her weekly hair appointments. All of us grandkids wanted to go on these trips so we would pile in her car to head to the salon, where we knew she would let us have twenty-five-cent Dr. Peppers out of the old glass dispenser. Every summer her stylist, Virginia, would tell me again that I had the same thick coarse hair as my grandma. I secretly loved the connection of our wild, unruly hair. On the way home, grandma would put one of us kids on her lap and let us drive the last couple blocks back to Edgewood. As we approached the house I would see the large cast-iron pots full of colorful flowers and smell the intoxicating scent of roses mixed with the entrancing magnolia and feel at peace.

My grandma Frances passed away at her home on May 31, 2004. I was fortunate enough to be present. I wouldn't say her death was peaceful. After months of fighting lung and brain cancer, chemo, radiation, and the side effects of prescription drugs, her final breaths were loud and labored. Her lungs no longer provided the vital exchange of oxygen and carbon dioxide necessary to sustain life.

The air was calm, as was the energy surrounding her body. Even my great-grandmother, who wept loudly at her bedside, had an aura of peace. Absolutely still, my mom and aunt stood by the bedroom door, reluctantly giving mother and daughter one last moment together. My sister and I lingered between the kitchen, hallway and bathroom, grief-stricken, holding our breaths while we waited for the end. The stillness that engulfed us is the universal life force, or Qi, that binds all life together.

Qi, the life-force energy that animates all living beings, is necessary for life. It is the guiding force behind all transformations of energy and connects us to the rest of the cosmos. It is Qi that creates all our homeostatic and metabolic reactions, the gas exchange in our lungs, and all the other vital functions of our body. With an abundance of Qi, there is vitality, good health, and a calm mind. Without enough Qi, disease or pain can arise, as blood and other necessary fluids are not distributed properly throughout the body. When we have depleted our Qi, and yin and yang separate, there is death. Death of the physical body is an absolute that none of us will escape, but that knowledge does not always prepare us for the loss of those we love the most.

After my grandma passed I went out in the yard to take refuge by the magnolia tree. Hearing her last difficult breaths, I felt incredibly and deeply grateful that my lungs still performed their essential function. I could smell the intoxicating fragrance of the magnolia flowers over the unmistakable stench of death that had permeated her home for days. Half-hiding behind the tree, I watched as my aunt Angela drove up and looked at me, and realizing she had missed the last few moments of her mothers life, ran into the house heavy with the desperation of grief. At that moment I bawled again and gave thanks to the universe for allowing me to be present and witness the passing of one of the most important people in my life.

At that moment of intense grief, I heard the magnolia sing to me, *Breathe life in, breathe life out. Transform anger into love, fear into courage and despair into growth.*

Evolution

Magnolia is one of our oldest flowering trees. Fossilized remains date the earliest magnolia to be from around a hundred million years ago. As the climate dramatically changed between 1.8 million and 11,000 years ago, the magnolias growing further south were spared from the last ice age. They thrived when many other species went extinct. The structure of the magnificent flowers and their strong carpels, which were originally pollinated by beetles, helped their evolution. Magnolia is a testament to nature's ability to adapt, survive and thrive.

Botanists and paleontologists first thought that some of the first flowers, like magnolia, were even larger and showier than they are today. Fossil evidence proves that they were wrong. Some of the first flowers were tiny, ranging from 0.04 to 0.23 inches in diameter. Gradually over time, they became larger, brighter, and more fragrant. Their vibrant colors of cream, pink and purple helped them stand out against all the green in the forest. Their scents enticed insects, and the bigger blossoms contained greater numbers of anthers, and therefore more pollen for distribution. Flowering plants evolved to be noticed and perpetuated.

Chinese Herbalism

Evidence shows that magnolia has been cultivated in Asia since the 7th century BC. The innate wisdom of magnolia is celebrated in classical China. The ancient story of *Mulan* is about compassionate action and familial duty. The warrior Mulan deceived everyone by claiming she was a man, but her actions were motivated by selfless action and love for her family and so she was ultimately forgiven. The main character Mulan and *Magnolia quinquepeta,* also called *Mu Lan,* are both associated with compassionate action and loyalty to yourself, your family and your community.

In Chinese medicine, *Mu Lan,* or the purple lily magnolia, can treat an imbalance of *Si Zhi Bu Ren* (Four Limbs Lack Compassion). *Si Zhi Bu Ren* is a weakness of the four limbs, with symptoms of fatigue, muscle atrophy and weakness of the extremities. Jeffrey Yuen, one of my favorite Daoist teachers, explains *Si Zhi Bu Ren* as a condition where one does not have the sense of priority of loyalty to himself, where one is not being true to one's values or beliefs. In essence, one is unable to stand up and act for what he believes in due to a weakness or deficit. I see a great need for us to use *Mu Lan* to help us be advocates and activists for the plants and the planet.

Another condition treated by *Mu Lan* is *Si Ji,* translated as dead flesh, which is an inability to support one's own weight or the weight of others. Someone with *Si Ji* is unable to take on any responsibilities. Physically they may fret or worry a lot, have poor digestion, or are unable to gain weight. Everyday obligations like paying bills are too much for someone with *Si Ji* to handle. Undernourished muscles and a lack of vitality are usually present in *Si Ji* as well. Due to a lack of transformative action in the middle *Jiao* (digestion), the Spleen's function of nourishing and stimulating tissue and muscle growth is blocked. If our muscles are literally weak from a lack of nutrients then it is easy to see why accepting responsibility or maturity is difficult or slowed.

In Chinese medicine, poor digestion and lack of nourishment are considered major factors in illness. The aromatic properties of Magnolia allow the person to open up enough to begin to transform and absorb the vital *Qi* that surrounds them. *Hou Po,* the bark of *Magnolia officinalis* twigs, has been used to treat the food stagnation that causes epigastric and abdominal fullness, distention, nausea and poor digestion. This stagnation is from a lack of responsibility to yourself and in the way you treat your body. With excessive intake of food, alcohol or fun, a state of stagnation occurs, which leads to poor digestion. Without proper assimilation of nutrients we can't nourish our muscles. The lack of muscle strength leads to the inability to stand up for ourselves and others.

Magnolia awakens us to the beauty and the responsibility of life. It also helps us transform these energies into useful bits of nutrients and intelligence. Once we are aware of the messages of magnolia, we can begin to transform this knowledge into vitality. There is a misunderstanding in healing or spiritual development where we think everyone should be able to buck up, be happy, let go and be enlightened. But from a Chinese medicine perspective, if we are unable to digest and transport what we ingest, we may not be able to reap the benefits of herbal medicine, meditation or acupuncture.

In my clinical practice I use magnolia to help the *Yi* (intellect) and the *Shen* (spirit). When the *Yi* and *Shen* are in balance this allows the Spleen to perform its duty of breaking down *Gu Qi* (food, drink, emotions) into vital substances, which are then transported to the tissues and muscles. When *Gu Qi* is transformed and properly assimilated there is more energy to put towards healing physically and spiritually. Magnolia, like all very aromatic plants, is about transformation. Think about how the aroma of magnolia creates an instant shift in mood and thought. It's hard to walk by a tree in bloom and not be captured by its intoxicating beauty.

Magnolia's Song

Turn to magnolia when you need support during times of transition like the death of a loved one, the end of a job or relationship, or when your child begins school. Magnolia is also useful when it is hard to digest things, be it food, information, or change. The beauty and aroma of magnolia can aid in transforming your life in ways unimaginable.

Breathe life in
Breathe life out
Transform hate into love
Fear into courage
Despair into growth

Magnolia Recipes

Magnolia Tea

- 3 grams dried *Hou Po* bark (*Magnolia officinalis*)
- 3-inch slice of fresh ginger root
- 1 slice dried licorice root

Simmer all ingredients for 15-20 minutes in 3 cups of water. Strain herbs and drink ½ cup of the warm tea before eating a heavy meal. The herbs will help break down and metabolize the food, eliminating distention, gas and bloating.

Mu Lan Oil

- Glass pint jar w/ lid
- Enough *Mu Lan* bark to fill the jar ¾ full
- Organic olive oil (or oil of choice)
- Cheesecloth or muslin
- Optional: add herbs like *Sang Ji Shen*, *Song Jie*, *Du Huo*, or any other herbs for muscle soreness and weakness.

Fill the glass jar ¾ full of *Mu Lan*. Cover the herbs with olive oil. Place cheesecloth or muslin between the jar and the lid and secure the lid tightly. Label the jar with the ingredient list and shake the jar gently. Infuse the herbs into the oil for 2-4 weeks, shaking daily. Keep the oil in a cool, dark place. Once the herbs have infused, strain out the herbs and put the infused oil in a dark glass container. Add essential oil and flower essence of magnolia if desired. Apply topically for sore, weak muscles or when you feel you need help standing up for something you know is right.

Breathe in Life Spritzer

- 6 drops magnolia flower essential oil
- 3 drops rose otto essential oil
- 1 drop vetiver essential oil

Mix the above essential oils into 2 ounces of carrier oil (olive, apricot kernel) and put into a 2-ounce spritzer bottle. Shake well and spritz yourself throughout the day. This is great for depression, to uplift the emotions and help transform and absorb the beauty of life.

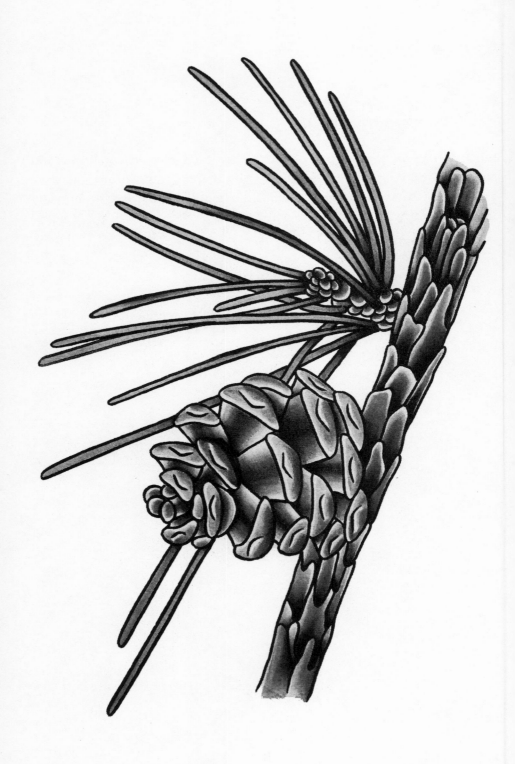

CHAPTER TWO

Pine: Grow Tall

Pinus tabulaeformis
Knotty Pine
Song Jie

>   **Properties**: Bitter, Warm
>   **Meridians entered**: Liver
>   **Elements influenced**: Wood
>   **Original habitat**: Northern China from Liaoning west to inner Mongolia, south to Shandong, Henan and Shaanxi; northern Korea; from an elevation of 100-2500 meters.
>   **Habitats**: Dry, sunny slopes at middle elevations.

Pinus longaeva
Bristlecone Pine

>   **Properties**: Bitter, Warm
>   **Meridians entered**: Lung
>   **Elements influenced**: Metal
>   **Original habitat**: High mountains from White and Inyo Mountains of CA, through southwestern and eastern Nevada, to central Utah at an elevation of 2134-3700 meters.
>   **Habitats**: Very dry, mid- to high-elevation exposed slopes and ridges; shade intolerant.

Pinus taeda
Loblolly Pine

> **Properties**: Bitter, Warm
> **Meridians entered**: Lung
> **Elements influenced**: Metal
> **Original habitat**: Flatlands to rolling hills from sea level to an elevation of 700 Meters.
> **Habitats**: From poorly drained to well-drained soil, usually on poor upland soils.

Description: There are around 120 species of conifers within the genus Pinus. Pine trees vary in size from 10 to 270 feet and can live to be thousands of years old. The branches, needles, and cones are in spiral arrangements and the bark of most pines is thick and scaly. The evergreen needles are the adult leaves, forming in the axil of the scale leaves. The cones are both male and female, with the female cone maturing between 1.5-3 years after pollination.

With suffering comes growth
Grow tall

Ancestral Medicine

Pine is the perfect example of how an injury can manifest into matter. Pine resin, sometimes called pitch, is released from deep within the cells of the tree when it has even a minute injury from a beetle or a branch break from the spring wind. The resin that comes from pine trees manifests in three different substances: volatile oil (known as turpentine), non-volatile rosin, and the high-boiling constituents with high odors and fixative values. When pine resin is burned these substances are evoked and the fragrance is released in its entirety. For centuries many cultures have burned pine and other resins in their religious rituals. The Mayans of Guatemala still burn pine resin in ceremonies.

My memories of pine are of both the sweet aroma in my neighborhood in Memphis, Tennessee as well as the putrid smell of the mills along our many highway drives. Many of my memories of pine are of me riding in the backseat of a car as we drove from one southern state to another, either for vacation or because we were moving again. "Pine in a line," my dad would say as we drove past acres of pine trees, which held the straight lines of timber that would all eventually end up in the pulp mills scattered throughout the South. Although for a few years I was "allergic" to pine pollen, I always loved the smell of pine trees. I didn't fully appreciate the magic and medicine pine provides until adulthood but I know its presence was pivotal in providing a sense of stability and familiarity in my young life of constant change.

My father's great-grandfather moved to Altha, Florida at the turn of the 19th century. He bought hundreds of acres of land and farmed many things, including sugarcane and pine trees. My grandfather and his slew of siblings eventually inherited the property and the land was subdivided amongst them. Most of what my family continued to grow was slash pine. Slash pine was known for its rapid growth and good heart timber, which forms when logs grow to over eighteen inches in width. But then the timber mills stopped accepting the older trees, insisting instead on the uniformity of sap timber, which are younger trees that rot without pressure treatment. Today there are three ages of pine trees on my granddad's land and I doubt it will ever be harvested for timber again.

I remember one year in the mid 1980's when my dad had to leave in a hurry to go down to Florida and help his family treat acres of bug-ridden pine trees to help save the rest of the trees for future harvest. They did not succeed and many acres were lost, along with thousands of dollars. It was then that I realized that for some, trees are commodities and their importance is defined by money, rather than necessity, beauty or grace. This realization made me sad. At this young age, my relationship with plants, and trees in particular, had been one of wonder, awe, and an almost Disney-like anthropomorphic view of nature. It seemed wrong that people could care for trees only for their monetary value. It still does.

It wasn't until a few years ago that I realized the importance of pine trees in the evolution of life on Earth. I never fathomed the immeasurable impact that pine and other ancient gymnosperms have had on all life that evolved afterward. The story of pine is a beautiful one—one that is nothing short of miraculous.

Evolution

Despite all of the diverse climates that have occurred since the Mesozoic period (245-65 million years ago), pine is one of the nine conifer families that have survived to modern times. Today we still have 105-125 species of pine trees in existence. To me, the diversity of humanity mirrors the diversity of pine trees. That we should be as unique and varied as one of our oldest ancestors is no coincidence. The resiliency in the genetic code of pines and their ability to adapt to extreme climactic change is an inspiration for our human adaptability as well. Pines and other conifers are also able to thrive in rocky, non-nutrient-rich soils. They are masters at conservation with their small, evergreen leaves.

A vital piece of conifer longevity is their symbiotic relationship with mycorrhiza, the beneficial type of fungi that grows in association with most plant roots, which allows for more surface area in root systems. The increase in surface area gives more water and nutrients to the tree. Mycorrhiza is an important reminder that we are integrally connected to a larger, unseen ecosystem. It is also a demonstration of how we are stronger when we build community.

Bristlecone pines are not only the oldest surviving pine species; some of them are the oldest living things on Earth. In the White Mountains of California, Methuselah, a 4600-year-old bristlecone pine, lives under the protection of the US Forest Service after an estimated 5000-year-old bristlecone was killed in 1964.

This act of violence was one of many that has inspired humans to act on behalf of species other than our own. The community of people who are actively working to save our old (or 2nd or 3rd-growth) forests is expanding. In the U.S., 90% of our virgin forests have been logged since 1600. In the Pacific Northwest, there are estimated to be only about two million acres left of our ancient forests, down from ten million acres in 1993— which, in turn, was a reduction from the 32.8 million acres recorded in the region between 1933 and 1945. We do not yet know the long-term impact of changing the ecosystem so drastically in such a short period of time.

Co-evolution

Pine is one of the most planted trees on the planet. In the last two hundred years, man has expanded the geographical area of the *Pinus* genus to the entire southern hemisphere. Unaided by man, this feat would have taken nature millions of years. We have a visceral connection to pine that makes our dependence on this plant very clear.

The evolution of early plant life and conifers in particular hold a very significant place in our human evolution. Without the presence of secondary metabolites (flavonoids, alkaloids, essential oils) our digestion and liver detoxification enzyme system would have evolved quite differently. By ingesting these plants, mammals developed sophisticated enzymatic processes to break down these otherwise toxic metabolites. It is worth noting that our migratory past also contributed to the development of these processes. Mammals had to adapt to new environments and food sources as they migrated and our physiology reflects that through our abilities to metabolize potentially toxic compounds.

Ancient & Modern Knowledge

The essential oil of pine is high in a-pinene and B-pinene, monoterpenes known to have analgesic and anti-inflammatory properties. They are also neurotonics, which help combat debility and fatigue. Pine is anti-infectious and is a powerful decongestant, like other aromatic plants. When inhaled, pine has an immediate effect on the limbic system, providing a regulatory effect on memory and sensory pathways.

In classical Chinese medicine, pine trees represent ancestral wisdom and longevity. Pine forests have been closely linked to sages and both embody refinement and virtue. Confucianism emphasizes respect for our ancestors and this has left many with resentment and shame if elders and ancestors are not treated properly. The medicine in pine trees can help resolve any bitterness we may have towards our ancestors and ourselves. Pine medicine helps us learn from the mistakes of our ancestors, allowing negativity and the emotions surrounding those mistakes to be forgiven, and then improving familial relations for future generations.

The views of our families and society can manifest in physical dis-ease if we absorb all the negativity others think about us. Our health can suffer further if we come to believe the things people think about us, or if we view ourselves as unworthy of love or acceptance. Even in modern China, people often put the wants of the family over their own desires for fear of dishonoring their family. It takes great courage to live out your Soul's desires and go against what society views as acceptable. Pine is that friend who awakens those desires and gives you the strength to stand tall in your convictions and actions.

Both pine cones and pine needles are used in Chinese medicine, but the most commonly used is the nodular branch of knotty pine (*Pinus tabulaeformis*), called *Song Jie*. *Song Jie* treats external injuries like sprains, strains and sore muscles from martial arts training or manual labor. *Bi Zheng*, or painful obstruction syndrome, is also treated with *Song Jie*-infused liquor. The warm, drying quality of *Song Jie* also alleviates the deep joint pain that is worse in cold, damp weather and makes flexion and movement difficult. This warming nature of *Song Jie* is unique, as many bitter herbs are cooling, and work to clear heat away with their cold temperatures. The warm nature of *Song Jie* brings heat to its high point, encouraging perspiration to begin to cool the body.

Knotty pine also treats boils and abscesses that appear on the face or head. These sores are thought to be from guilt, especially in regards to your relationship to yourself and your family. Pine is your ally when there is a mal-alignment between you and society or your family. There are times when you need to break away from what the majority of people hold in popular belief. Pine is your ally to get you in alignment with yourself. Pine allows you to accept yourself when others cannot understand or support your decision to live your truth.

We now know that trauma from one generation can transmit to the next, not only in patterns of behavior, but also in DNA. The positive thing is that we are also discovering that we can spiritually break patterns of trauma—and even transform cellular DNA. There is a whole new branch of science called behavioral epigenetics that studies the changes in organisms caused by the modification of gene expression rather than the alteration of the genetic code itself.

One such study examined the glucocorticoid steroid receptors in rats. Scientists discovered that rats who were neglected by their mothers had highly methylated receptors, whereas rats who got plenty of attention from their mothers had receptors that were rarely methylated. The rats with the highly methylated receptors were less attentive mothers, in turn, and passed that gene down to their offspring. But when rats born of neglected mothers were given to attentive mothers, they developed less methylation and did not pass the methylated genes on to their offspring.

Another study compared the brains of suicide victims with the brains of those who died of other causes. Genes of the hippocampuses of those who died by suicide were methylated, while the other brains were not. In the brains of those who were abused as children, there were even higher rates of methylation in the hippocampus. Similarly, blood samples of Russian children in orphanages were found to have more methylated genes than the blood samples of children raised by their biological parents (Discover Magazine, May 2013).

This methylation occurred in genes that play an important role in neural communication and brain function and development, which could partially explain why some people are more prone to depression or suicide. In such people, development and communication are stunted and further insulated by an extra methyl layer, resulting in an inability to fully love themselves or others.

Pine's Song

I don't know about pine and its ability to reduce methylation, but I do know it is used to heal ancestral trauma. It is the plant that sees you for who you are and honors that by helping you see it in yourself. As an herbalist, I think of the other herbs that open our hearts to reveal the beauty we have inside: rose, hawthorn, magnolia, and pine. Pine also gives you the strength to see through the lies you've been told and have told yourself. Pine helps you stand up for your beliefs and advocate for yourself. Pine helps you adapt and grow.

With suffering comes growth
Grow tall

Pine Recipes

Song Jie Oil

- 30 grams *Song Jie* (nodular branch of knotty pine)
- 500 ml vodka, gin or liquor of choice

Pound and grind knotty pine into powder, and then soak it in alcohol for seven days in a glass jar. Shake the container once daily while soaking. Strain out herbs and store extract in a glass bottle. Take 15 ml (1 tablespoon) twice daily for arthralgia or rheumatic arthritis.

Healthy Lung Diffuser

- 2 drops peppermint essential oil
- 2 drops pine essential oil
- 2 drops eucalyptus essential oil
- 2 drops lavender essential oil
- 1 drop thyme essential oil

Bring 4 cups water to a boil. Turn off heat and add essential oils. Cover head and bowl with a towel and inhale deeply to open nasal passages.

Pine Pitch Balm

- One quarter-size piece of pine pitch (According to Theophrastus, the purest pitch is obtained from trees growing in a sunny, north-facing position.)
- 4 ounces apricot kernel oil (preferably infused with pine needles)
- 1/2 ounce beeswax

Place pine pitch, oil and beeswax over a double boiler and gently warm over low heat until the beeswax and pine pitch melt. Remove from heat and pour into a 4-ounce glass jar. Do not put on lid until completely solid. The balm can be applied to the chest for congestion or to sore, achy muscles. For a more spiritual use of the balm, add to the area of your third eye and the soles of your feet to help you stand tall in your convictions.

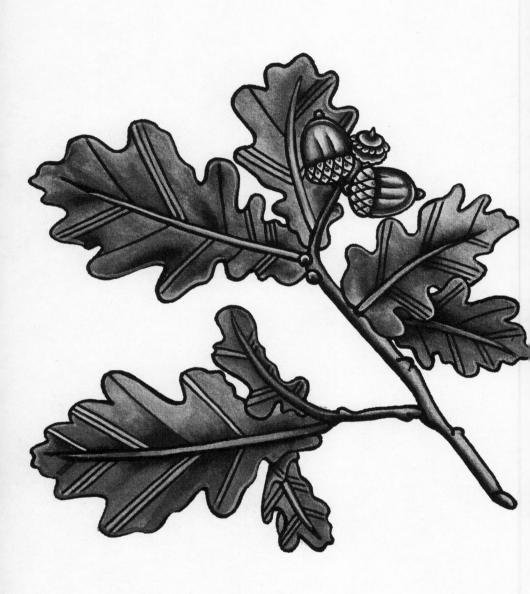

CHAPTER THREE

Oak: Be Strong, Be Resilient, Be Wise

Quercus fusiformis
Plateau Oak

Taste: Bitter, Slightly Aromatic
Temperature: Warm
Meridians Entered: Lung, Large Intestine
Natural Habitat: Native range includes the Quartz Mountains and Wichita Mountains in Oklahoma, through Texas, to the Mexican states of Coahuila, Tamaulipas, and Nuevo Leon.

Description: There are over 600 species of oak, each with their own distinct qualities and habitats. Oaks can grow to 100 feet or more. Some trees are deciduous, others evergreen, and some are semi-evergreen. Oaks produce a fruit called acorns that take 6-18 months to mature. The leaves are spirally arranged and can be serrated or lobed. Oak trees can live to be over 1,000 years old.

> ***Be strong***
> ***Be resilient***
> ***Be wise***

Ancestral Medicine

I lived in Lubbock, Texas between the ages of eight and twelve. My friend and neighbor had a beautiful oak tree that took up her entire front yard. After school and on weekends, she and I spent hours playing in the branches, making up stories about nature spirits and dreaming about what we would do when we were adults. Her family had another house in the country, so I have many memories of being in the tree by myself, retreating to it when I needed to be alone.

As the perpetual new kid, there was always an awkward period as I transitioned from one school to another. During that transition, the oak tree was a retreat for my soul and my imagination. Spirits of adventure inhabited those branches and I would converse with the insects and birds, none of whom ever asked or cared where I came from. I would climb the tree and daydream, imagining a life as stable as the branch I sat upon. Little did I know, the oak tree was infusing me with the strength and courage I needed to adapt to persistent change.

I was in the sixth grade when my first childhood friend died. David Lawrence was two years older than I was and lived near my family in Trenton, Georgia. He was one of the people I had known since I was a small child, one of the few constants I had when I'd visit family in the summer and on holidays. After hearing that David had died of unknown causes (later we would find out it was undiagnosed Type 1 diabetes), I climbed to the highest branch of that oak tree and cried, allowing the strength of the branches to hold me as I howled with a sadness I couldn't control. I already had a morbid association with death—my sister's Type 1 diabetes and my own ureter reflux surgery that hospitalized me for two weeks still affected my psyche. Crying until exhausted, I completely let go and allowed myself to relax against the large trunk. I felt an odd sense of guilt for being alive, for enjoying the breeze on my wet face as I looked back at my house next door. I was disoriented from the emotions but profoundly calm, and I felt an arcane need to understand what death really was.

Global Knowledge

With a lifespan of over 200 years, it is no surprise that oaks are also symbols of fertility, longevity and protection. Acorns are worn as fertility amulets and are carried to preserve youthfulness and health. Some Wiccan traditions used an oak wand topped with an acorn to conduct fertility magic. We know that the Druids held their sacred ceremonies in oak groves, where Pliny witnessed them accessing the insights of the universe as they held their sacred rites among the old wise trees.

Oak trees have been a source of sustenance and protection for thousands of years. The oldest evidence of a human settlement with oak trees is from the Jordan Valley and dates back over 20,000 years. With over 400 species of oak trees that thrive from the Mediterranean to subtropical rainforest, it is no wonder that so many cultures look at these beings with reverence and awe. Oaks not only provide a highly nutritious, abundant food source for animals, they are a keystone species, meaning that entire ecosystems depend upon them for survival.

All around the world, since the beginning of humanity, people have relied on acorns as a staple part of their diets. First, however, we had to develop a careful procedure for making them edible. After being soaked overnight, their shells would be split open and the kernels were spread on open baskets to dry. Once dry, they were ground to flour in a stone mortar, and then leached over a frame of incense cedar twigs repeatedly until the acorn meal turned pink, indicating the tannins had been removed. The meal could then be baked into bread or made into soup, providing much-needed protein, amino acids and essential nutrients. The gathering and preparation of acorns is a long-held tradition that has brought people together and sustained communities around the world.

Keystone Species

Jolie Elan of the Go Wild Institute talks about legends that foretold how our precious relations in nature would disappear if we stop caring for them. She sees this as true with the decline of keystone species like salmon, whales, and oaks. California oaks and tan oaks are infested with sudden oak death and keystone species around the world are in decline. Jolie believes that in order to keep ecosystems intact, sustainability and environmental education are important but insufficient. She sees ceremony as a necessary component of honoring our plant relations. When we gather in the groves and share songs and recipes about oaks, they thrive with our reverence for their rightful place as the providers and protectors of the ecosystem. The diversity and vitality of our planet depend on the health of our keystone species. The health of the planet depends on the health of the people. Just as it has been for thousands of years, people need the medicine of oak.

Traditional Herbalism

In folklore, oaks signify strength and resiliency. An oak tree can be struck by lightning and continue to stand tall and strong, providing protection for the numerous species that settle near their groves. Oaks can also sprout from damaged trunks, forming natural coppices. After forest fires oaks send out shoots that produce clones of the parent tree. Long associated with Thor, the Norse god of thunder, lightning and war, the strength of oak has been connected with warriors and soldiers and the strength needed to survive the traumas of war. The essence of oak tree has been used by some practitioners for combat veterans, for those exhausted warriors who continue to fight long after the wars are over. Oak essence has also been useful in reducing the fear and anxiety associated with trauma. Emotional scars run deeper than physical scars and the vibrational medicine of oak essences are subtle enough to travel into our most intimate wounds.

The medicinal actions of oak bark are astringent and antiseptic. Used to tan animal hides, the bark can also treat weeping sores and dermatitis. Hippocrates used the fumes of oak leaves to calm women who had hysteria. Galen, a prominent Greek physician and philosopher who lived between 130 and 210 AD, later applied bruised oak leaves to acute wounds.

The oaks' astringency was not only known in medicine, but also to those who ate the acorns. This is why such an elaborate process of leaching and grinding was needed to make most acorns palatable. Acorn preparation yielded other benefits, too. There are accounts of a penicillin-like mold that was made by covering the acorn meal to make it sweat and mold. The skin of the mold was peeled off and kept in a damp place, and then when needed was applied to boils or infected sores to draw out the infection. A wash of oak bark can help with weepy, irritated skin from eczema, psoriasis or poison oak. Oak can be the first line of defense against external pathogens and is good for those who contract colds and flus easily. In Chinese medicine we called this pattern, *Wei Qi Xu*, a deficiency of the defensive *Qi*. *Wei Qi Xu* can manifest in different ways, depending on the constitution of the patient. Those with a deficiency of the defensive *Qi* may also have seasonal allergies, asthma, and eczema. When people with deficient constitutions get an external cold or flu, they may sweat profusely. A tea of oak bark can strengthen the *Wei Qi* and stop the perspiration, which is important because the loss of fluids can lead to *yin* deficiency. Use oak bark to fortify and armor against external influences. Oak consolidates and tones, creating a container for essence and matter to transform without leakage.

The Balance of Life

For millennia, oaks have been used and worshipped for their life-giving properties. As we spend time in their groves we are reminded of how vital they are to their environment. Squirrels scamper and birds nest in their branches as a slew of insects and larvae house immeasurable life, all of which contributes much more than we know to this delicate balance. We take the intricacy of nature for granted and it is time we remember our survival depends on mycorrhizae, bacteria and microorganisms we haven't even discovered yet. Their survival depends on us finding some coherent balance between co-existing on this planet and destroying entire ecosystems.

The way we live on this planet is not sustainable. Mass consumerism as we know it can not continue if we wish to have renewable resources left over the next seven generations. The environmental devastation over the last hundred years is mind-blowing. We all play a role in that destruction as we consume resources daily with electricity, fuel and food. Our most cherished habits come great distances to conveniently appear on our shelves: coffee, tea, coconut oil, and tropical fruit. The list is endless, as is human consumption.

Paradigm shifts do not come easily. The death of mass consumerism is going to shatter illusions that have been perpetuated for the last few hundred years. There will be resistance but once we begin to listen to our plant relations we will see that our only way to thrive as a species on this planet is to stop the insanity of consumerism. We are resilient and will adapt to this reality. As we return to nature, the segment of our identity we define through consumerism will fade and an older part will awaken, enlivening a matrix of connections older than civilization.

Oak's Song

Oak is here to protect you and guard you from those who would attack you for your beliefs and rituals. Oak provides much-needed nourishment and sustenance along your journey to the truth. Oak gives you strength when you don't feel you can carry on.

> *Be strong*
> *Be resilient*
> *Be wise*

Oak Recipes

Oak Bark Skin Wash

Fill large muslin teabag 3/4 full with equal parts dried: oak bark, calendula flowers, prunella flowers, plantain leaves. Use as a washcloth in the shower or place teabag in a bath to reduce inflammation from weepy, irritated skin.

Acorn Crackers

Mix 1 cup acorn flour (directions in chapter), 1 cup all-purpose flour, 2 tbsp. sugar, 1 tsp. salt. Cut in 2 tbsp. vegetable shortening or butter and add enough water to make into a soft dough. Knead gently. Place onto a large floured cutting board, cover, and let sit for 10 minutes. Roll dough with a floured rolling pin until about 1/8" thick. Prick surface of dough with a fork. Add sesame, hemp, or sunflower seeds. Cut into rectangles and place on ungreased cookie sheet. Bake at 350 degrees for 20-30 minutes. Let cool and store in a glass container. Makes 2-3 dozen crackers.

Survive & Thrive Essence

In a crystal or glass bowl, add 8 ounces of spring water. Take bowl down to the oak grove and sit quietly for a few minutes. Ask permission to take parts of the tree for medicine. Once given permission, take a small amount of five parts of the tree: leaf, bark, twig, flower, acorn. If there is exposed root, take a very small piece without injuring the tree. Allow tree parts to infuse in the water for three days. Strain off plant material and collect water in an 8-ounce glass bottle. Take 1-7 drops of the oak essence as needed for mental or physical stamina and strength.

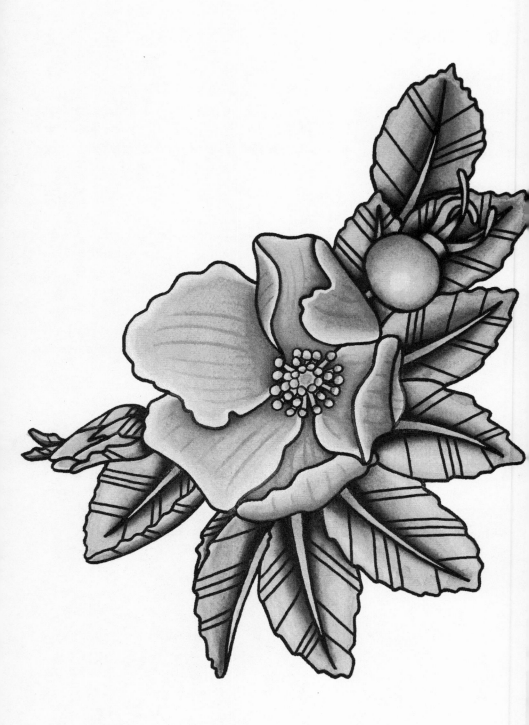

CHAPTER FOUR

Rose: Love Yourself Every Day

Rosa rugosa
Rose
Mei Gui Hua

- **Properties:** Sweet, Slightly Bitter, Warm
- **Meridians entered:** Liver, Spleen
- **Original habitat:** On the coast of northeastern China, Japan, Korea and southeastern Siberia.
- **Habitats:** Now cultivated and naturalized in much of the world.

Rosa chinensis
Rose
Yue Ji Hua

- **Properties:** Sweet, Warm
- **Meridians entered:** Liver
- **Original habitat:** Southwest China, in Guizhou, Hubei, and Sichuan provinces.
- **Habitats:** Used for breeding of many modern garden roses; hybrids are now grown around the world.

Rosa laevigata
Rosehip
Jin Ying Zi

- **Properties:** Sour, Neutral
- **Meridians entered:** Kidney, Urinary Bladder, Large Intestine
- **Original Habitat:** Southern China, Laos, Vietnam
- **Habitats:** Considered invasive in many places, including the United States.

Description: True roses usually compound leaves with an odd number of leaflets and prickles (not thorns) along the stem. The flowers are often fragrant, 5-petaled, and produce a hip as the fruit type. Most of the roses grown in gardens are hybrids, with varied petal numbers, aroma, and thorns.

Love yourself
Every day

Traditional Herbalism

I doubt there has ever been a flower so revered as rose. Prior to modern hybridization, there were about 250 species of rose. Within two hundred years, there were thousands of rose varieties as the popularity of rose grew with the help of Empress Josephine, Queen of Flowers. Some of the earliest written records of rose are Homer's allusions to them in the *Iliad* and *Odyssey*. Poems to rose date back as early as 600BC. A Hindu god, Vishnu, formed Lakshmi from 108 large and 1,008 small roses, making them an early symbol of beauty.

The delicate fragrance of rose has been captured as rosewater for millennia. The production of rose water in Iran dates back at least 2,500 years. Historical exploration shows ancient Egyptians and Greeks extolling the spiritual and medicinal virtues of roses in their art, music and writings. Poetry, paintings and horticulture have all contributed to humanity's awe and obsession with the mighty rose.

Rose petals have been in most pharmacopeias across the globe and are recognized for their tonic and cooling properties. Since antiquity, medicinal and food preparations have been made with whatever rose species people had access to. Even today, roses are bred for their fragrance and beauty, and are still used in food and medicinal products around the world.

John Gerard recorded many of the ideas of the Greek physician and botanist Pedanius Dioscorides, and other notable herbalists, in 1636. Gerard's love of roses is evident in his three-volume *General Historie of Plants*, where he states "*...for the Rose doth deserve the chief and prime place among all floures whatsoever.*" Gerard includes a poem to rose from Greek poet Anacreon Thius:

> The Rose is the honour and beauty of floures,
> The Rose in the care and love of the Spring:
> The Rose is the pleasure of th' heavenly Pow'rs.
> The boy of faire Venus, Cythera's Darling,
> Doth wrap his head round with garlands of Rose,
> When to the dances of the Graces he goes.

In Greek antiquity, rose was used as both a wound antidote and as an eye makeup. Dioscorides gives recipes for rose salves and liquids for the eyes, ears, gums and intestines. Several roses are listed in Dioscorides' *Materia Medica*, including common garden varieties, wild rose, and a variety without prickles that had not yet made it to London, where Gerard was writing. The distilled water of rose was used to refresh the spirits, strengthen the heart, and for all conditions that required gentle cooling. The fragrance of rose can bring on a restful sleep.

Nicholas Culpeper, a 17th-century English herbalist, could not say enough about the rose and he writes about several things rose is good for. Not to understate the important role rose plays in herbalism, he states, "To write at large of every one of these, would make my book swell too big, it being sufficient for a volume of itself, to speak fully of them." Several preparations he does mention are distilled water of roses, vinegar of roses, rose ointment, oils of rose, rose conserve, sugar of roses, syrup of dried roses and honey of roses. Culpeper distinguishes between red and white roses by saying the white rose is more cooling and binding than the red rose, especially those that are not fully open yet. He says fresh rose is more bitter and can purge the humors. Dried roses have a more binding and astringent quality.

Chinese Herbalism

In Chinese herbalism, we use three different varieties of roses. *Rosa rugosa*, or *Mei Gui Hua*, translated as "beautiful flower," relieves *Qi* constraint and stagnation and can reduce the stifling feeling in the chest and abdomen that occurs with stress or emotions. *Mei Gui Hua* promotes the movement of *Qi*, harmonizes blood, and disperses blood stasis. *R. rugosa* can also regulate menstruation, reduce the menstrual pain associated with blood stasis, and alleviate the symptoms of PMS, including breast tenderness, depression and anxiety.

Rosa chinensis, or *Yue Ji Hua*—"moon season flower"—is sweet and warm. It is traditionally used to invigorate blood and regulate menses. Cooked with brown sugar, *Yue Ji Hua* treats scanty menstruation and the associated abdominal pain, constipation, and emotional distress. Scrofula can be treated with a formula of *Yue Ji Hua, Xia Ku Cao (Prunella vulgaris), Bei Mu (Fritillaria cirrhosa),* and *Mu Li (Concha Ostreae).* Moon season flower is not used during pregnancy because it invigorates blood. Those with Spleen or Stomach *Qi* deficiency may have diarrhea with excessive use.

The fruit of *Rosa laevigata, Jin Ying Zi,* or "golden cherry fruit," is sour, astringent and neutral. *Jin Ying Zi* stabilizes the energy of the kidneys and retains the vital essence that is lost during involuntary ejaculation, urinary incontinence and vaginal discharge. The astringent action associated with the sour flavor can help with rectal and uterine prolapse and can help stop excessive uterine bleeding or chronic diarrhea. The astringent quality of *Jin Ying Zi* helps us retain our vital essences, which contribute to longevity and the stability of our thoughts and emotions.

Medicine of Love

Rose is engrained in our collective memory as a flower associated with love. Most of the time we take this to mean an expression of love towards another person. The medicine of rose is that it helps you to love yourself too. Once you love yourself as eagerly as you love others, deep healing occurs.

Since childhood I have found it extremely difficult to love myself. I would blame myself for being ugly and awkward and there were times I didn't know if I would ever like myself. No amount of love from my parents could stop me from thinking that I was unworthy of love. I was uncomfortable in my body and wondered if I would ever be happy. I wanted to love myself but couldn't find a way.

My clinical work has given me the perspective that everybody could use a little more self-love. Even those who appear overly confident or superior need to love themselves. They actually need it even more than those delicate souls whom we feel the need to care for or protect. Rose will help soften these overconfident people, allowing them to see themselves entirely and love themselves for their weaknesses and not just their strengths. Rose will help them accept themselves for who they truly are and not only for what they accomplish.

When you really allow rose to enter your heart, the work is subtle yet deeply insightful. At first, just enjoy the aroma. Then allow the images to come. Once the images clear, let the emotions come. Either immense happiness or a deep sadness that has been latent may come to the surface and release. The release is cathartic but also soothing, like the arm of a friend draped over you, holding you tight through your despair. This is rose. Rose is here to help you let go of the hurt and just love yourself.

One of my personal experiences with rose came with the inhalation of rose essential oil. I was feeling intensely sad on the day before the anniversary of my friend Chachi's suicide. On this day I was having trouble wrapping my head around how she could end her existence in this life. I was weepy and disoriented, my mind and spirit unsettled. I applied a single drop of rose essential oil to my chest and forehead and put one drop into my diffuser. Initially I got a little mentally irritated—which is not my usual response to rose—and my body was not responding with the peace and relaxation rose usually brings. For the first time in my life, rose was not comforting, but was overwhelming and almost nauseating. Getting more anxious by the moment, I turned off the diffuser and filled my day with work and domestic chores. That night I slept soundly but when I awoke my jaw felt like I'd been clenching it all night. I had a headache and was feeling disconnected and all out of sorts.

As the morning passed I couldn't escape thoughts of Chachi and I realized I had been struggling all night with what she had done to herself. I couldn't believe she would destroy her beautiful, kind soul. The despair and desperation she must have felt in that moment had been rattling me for months.

The death or separation of any loved one is extremely difficult. When someone takes their own life, there is a visceral reaction, as well as an emotional one. Something deep within our DNA revolts against the killing of itself. Everything in our nature is designed to sustain our own life, not destroy it. We feel the loss from suicide, right down to our core. As soon as I let myself be with the anguish I felt, a downpour of tears erupted from a place deep within my heart where I had been stuffing my shock, grief and despair over the past year. I turned back on the diffuser with rose essential oil and added lavender, hoping it would give me the relaxation I needed to accompany the release that rose had facilitated. The lavender brought me a noticeable sense of peace and the calmness I was having trouble obtaining. I felt immense love and compassion for myself. I made a vow to love myself every day, so that I wouldn't forget how precious I am. I began to take my first deep breaths in days.

Rose's Song

Rose allows you to open your heart and gives you the strength to release any suppressed grief, anxiety, or fear. If the thought of opening your heart to acceptance or forgiveness makes you feel weak or vulnerable, envision a barrier of thorny rose bushes encircling you. The aroma and beauty of the roses will awaken and soothe you, while the thorns protect you from anything that surfaces in your release. Call on rose when you begin to doubt your magnificence, criticize yourself or others, feel blue, or just need a little more joy in your life.

Love yourself
Every day

Rose Recipes

A note on using roses: Roses and other cut flowers are commonly sprayed with several chemicals and pesticides. Make sure you only use organic or non-sprayed flowers.

I Nourish My Soul Oil

In a 1-ounce glass bottle add 3 drops rose essential oil, 1 drop vanilla absolute, 2 drops frankincense essential oil and 2 drops vetiver essential oil to 1 ounce apricot kernel oil. Shake well. Anoint yourself with the fragrant oil as needed for meditation, relaxation or a reminder to love yourself.

Fragrant Flower Tea

Harvest a handful of roses, daisies, calendula, violet flowers and any other edible flower. (If using lavender, use only a small amount, as it can taste soapy.) Pour hot water over flowers and cover completely. Steep for 20 minutes in a glass jar with lid on. Strain flowers and collect water in a glass quart jar. Drink the tea throughout the day to open your heart and promote relaxation.

Rose Petal Wine

- 1/2 cup dried Rose petals
- 1/2 cup honey
- 1 liter white wine

Steep rose petals and honey in wine for 2 weeks. Shake daily. Strain out petals and collect wine in a dark glass bottle. Sip an ounce or two of wine nightly or add to hot water as an instant tea.

PART II

Adolescence/Realizations

Honeysuckle, Tea, Tobacco, Cannabis

Oh, adolescence. There is nothing more confusing, irritating, and exhilarating than our pubescent years. This is when my rebellion and search for my own personal truth began. I was no longer the lonely, innocent little girl. By the time I was nine, I had been through serious medical conditions like scarlet fever, chronic urinary tract infections, and ureter-reflux surgery. I had moved to more places than some people would in their entire life. The feelings of angst, insecurity, and fear were permeating deeper and I began to look for outside influences to fill the gaping holes inside. Music and friends helped, but I felt even more disconnected from everyone around me.

For Part II I chose Honeysuckle, for the loss of innocence of youth; Tea, for my longing for community; Tobacco, for my rebellious spirit; and Cannabis, for my awakening.

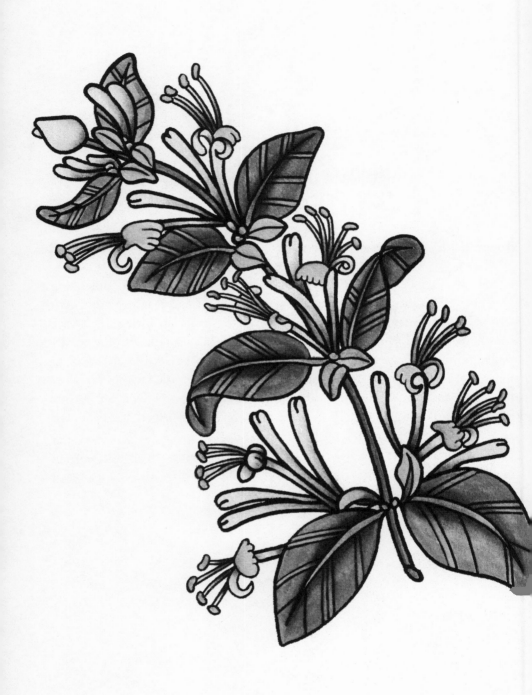

CHAPTER FIVE

Honeysuckle: Dissolve & Evolve

Lonicera japonica
Honeysuckle
Jin Yin Hua

Properties: Sweet, Cold
Meridians entered: Lung, Stomach, Large Intestine
Elements influenced: Metal, Earth
Original habitat: Eastern Asia
Habitats: Highly invasive; takes over wherever it is planted.

Description: Honeysuckle is a deciduous, sometimes semi-evergreen, twining vine that can grow up to 30 feet. The leaves are oval and dark green. The fragrant, two-lipped, tubular flowers are white that fade to yellow. The berries are small and black.

Dissolve and evolve

Innocence

I can still smell the honeysuckle of my childhood. In the summer in the South there are days of stifling heat when the humidity and the temperature both hover around a hundred and you can't even move without sweat pouring down your body. The only reward for this stickiness is the aromatic nectar that also oozes out of the honeysuckle flowers. On these days, the honeysuckle drops are as thick as the air, as the syrup intensifies with the rising humidity. Each flower gives one drop of sugary nectar if you delicately pull on the stamen and stop right before you pull the head out. One deliciously aromatic drop of essence that dissolves instantly on your tongue is the reward for your delicate grace. If you've ever had this experience, you know it's worth it.

Many people see honeysuckle as an extremely invasive plant that will take over any fence line or building it finds. I see honeysuckle as a reminder of how exquisite we are. The sensual nature of honeysuckle is evident in its alluring aroma and its propensity for reproducing itself. I believe this invasive climber has deliberate reasons for spreading herself so widely. Honeysuckle reminds us of the purity of our true essences. Like this tenacious vine, we are ambrosia to the core. I have very fond childhood memories of extracting the nectar from the flower and experiencing the way just one drop of its sweetness could arouse desires deep within me.

I remember one exceptionally hot, humid day when I was ten. My older sister Lia and I were in someone's backyard, attempting to extract the nectar from the vine that was taking over the fence. After many unsuccessful tries and a few successful ones, Lia got bored and walked away. I remained, unsatisfied with my attempts, as I had not yet attained one as sweet as I knew possible. I looked over all the flowers and picked one that I thought would be the peak of ripeness. Slowly and systematically I extracted the single bead, brought it to my lips, and sucked slowly to inhale both the aroma and the sugar. At the moment the nectar dissolved, I had a vision of myself as a very young child. I was at a honeysuckle vine, in ecstasy, as I tasted each flower I could reach, searching for that perfect drop. I laughed and dissolved into the freedom and innocence of youth. I wouldn't feel that way again for a long time.

Traditional Herbalism

In *Gerard's Herbal* (also called *The General History of Plants*), the most widely circulated English-language botanical reference in the 17ᵗʰ century, John Gerard describes a treatment wherein honeysuckle flowers are steeped in oil and set in the sun to be used as an anointment for a body that is very cold and numb. As an herb that can cool the body, it is the act of steeping honeysuckle in the sun that gives it a warming quality. Gerard is probably referring to cold, numb limbs from arthritis or being in a cold environment, but what if we expand that to mean a cold, numb personality? Might such people also benefit from an ointment that can warm their cold hearts? As an Aquarius who becomes cold, numb, and emotionally detached as a defense mechanism, I know honeysuckle can dissolve the thickest layer of ice surrounding a wounded heart. Honeysuckle has cracked me open more than once, intoxicating me with sweetness, forcing me to look deep within myself, to find the love and connection that was elusive most of my childhood.

Although I did keep some pen pals for most of my youth, moving around a lot did not help me to solidify long-term relationships. I also felt insecure and awkward with my short hair and was mistaken for a boy more than once. Once when I was eleven, a girl asked me to slow skate because she thought I was a boy. I should have been flattered because she was pretty, and she thought I was cute and a good skater. Instead, I was humiliated. I was already grappling with what it meant to be a woman, having recently started my menstrual cycle. Insecurities about my body rapidly developed and worsened my self-confidence further.

Overnight, it seemed, I developed breasts. My hair was still short, but there was now no denying what sex I was. I could feel hormonal shifts as my body grew and bled. I had sensual thoughts and urges about boys at school, the young GIs I saw on the base, and the rock stars I saw on MTV. I noticed the ways guys looked at my chest and I knew I looked older than most of the other girls my age. I still felt awkward and timid, and now my changing body was bringing me further unwanted attention.

As it is with many people, every rejection, criticism or disgrace was fodder for the flames of self-hatred for me. I was smart but not pretty. I had big breasts and thought I was fat. Some of this I believed, but a lot of it came from others. Boys snapped my bra and made fun of my chest at school and so I did my best to hide them. The girls were cliquish and alienated me for my differences. Grown men would compare me to my older sister, who was becoming a beautiful young woman, thin-framed with long blond hair. I didn't want to tell my friends how confused and afraid I was of all the changes in my body. I filled myself with judgment and blame until I began to become an angry person. I know teenagers are known for their anger and erratic behavior, but a lot of my youthful angst was due to how I felt about myself. These emotions filled me up and came spewing out as cynicism and rebellion against the world.

Chinese Herbalism

In Chinese medicine, honeysuckle is called *Jin Yin Hua,* or golden silver flower, and as a flowering vine, it is seen as delicate, extremely beautiful and aromatic. According to Chinese herbals it is a very strong herb that can clear heat from the body. Along with clearing heat, honeysuckle also dissolves phlegm and opens the sinuses, making it one of the best herbs for sinus infections where there is yellow, sticky phlegm. Honeysuckle treats what is called summer heat, which is when you have a fever and a heavy sensation from getting overheated, which can lead to heat stroke.

Honeysuckle also treats heat in the *Qi* level. When heat is in the *Qi* level, we describe it as the "Four Bigs": high fever, high thirst, heavy sweating, and a forceful pulse. In herbalism, when there is heat in the *Qi* level, we treat it with an herb with a cold nature to drive the heat out of the body. Once the heat is gone, we usually stop using or reduce the cold herb to protect digestion.

Honeysuckle is cold enough to drive heat out of the body and also to eliminate toxins. Honeysuckle, taken both internally and externally, can treat sores and abscesses that arise from toxic heat. Since it has an affinity for the stomach and intestines, honeysuckle can also help reduce the dysentery and diarrhea caused by toxicity. It's interesting to me that so many beautifully aromatic plants, like honeysuckle, also have very strong broad-spectrum antibiotic and anti-inflammatory properties, which can rid the body of toxicity.

I believe the energy of honeysuckle, with its alluring aroma and strong therapeutic effects, can also clear toxic or abusive relationships out of one's life. Honeysuckle medicine reminds us that we don't deserve or need that toxicity in our life. It's as if the aroma of honeysuckle makes it so we see our self-worth and the divinity within ourselves that deserves love and acceptance. When I meditate with honeysuckle, I see my own magnificence reflected in the beauty and strength of the golden silver flowers.

In Chinese medicine we know that excess emotions can create turbidity and toxicity within the body, mind and spirit. The aromatic quality of the flowers encourages the transformation of dense energies, like anger and grief. Once transformed into lighter vibrations of compassion and acceptance, greater healing can occur. Honeysuckle can clear out muddled thoughts and emotions that make our spirits feel heavy. When we gain more clarity, latent memories, emotions, and desires awaken. Stirring up these experiences can be frightening, but it is one of the first steps to healing. Once you are able to remember what your authentic spirit truly desires, you are on the path back home.

Honeysuckle is your ally to remind yourself that you are worthy and capable of accepting divine love and compassion. It is when we can dissolve into the discernment of our own hearts that we evolve into the people we long to be.

Honeysuckle's Song

Honeysuckle bears witness to your grace and reflects that grace back to you. Allow yourself to dissolve into the beautiful mystery that is you.

Dissolve and evolve

Honeysuckle Recipes

Honeysuckle Honey

- 1 cup fresh honeysuckle flowers (Make sure they are not sprayed with pesticides.)
- 2 cups honey

Place honey and flowers in the top of a double boiler and heat on low for 20-30 minutes. Turn off heat and strain out flowers. Store honey in a glass jar. Add a teaspoon to black or herbal tea.

Fresh Honeysuckle Tea

Gather a handful of fresh honeysuckle flowers. Boil 2 cups of water. Pour hot water over flowers. Cover cup with lid. Steep for 10 minutes. Strain out flowers and compost plant material. Slowly drink the fragrant tea. Sweeten tea with honeysuckle honey.

Sweet & Spicy Sinus Steam

Collect a handful of the following fresh herbs: honeysuckle, rosemary, thyme, holy basil, eucalyptus leaves, or any aromatic herbs you have growing around you. Place fresh herbs in a bowl of hot steaming water. Cover your head with a towel and hover above bowl. Inhale deeply for 5-10 minutes to open clogged sinuses.

Honeysuckle Meditation

Allow yourself to go back to a moment when you carefully extracted nectar from a honeysuckle flower. Re-experience the sweetness of that one moment in time.

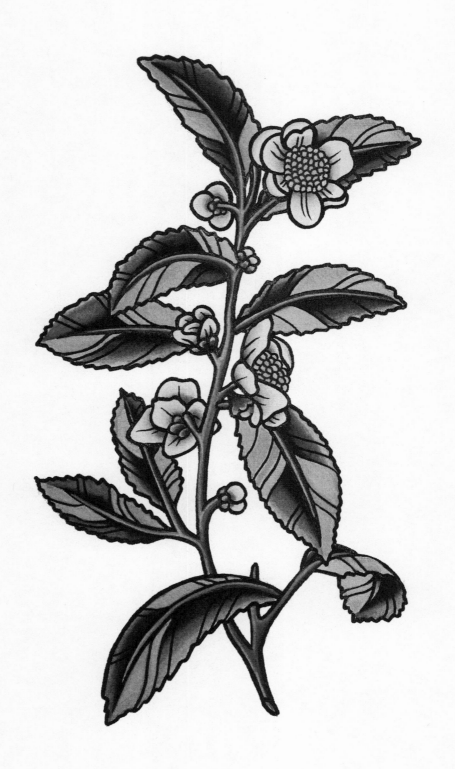

CHAPTER SIX

Tea: Gather Together

Camellia sinensis
Tea
Lu Cha

- **Taste:** Bitter, Sweet
- **Temperature:** Cool (white and green), Warm (black and puer)
- **Meridians entered:** Heart, Stomach
- **Elements influenced:** Fire, Earth
- **Original habitat:** Southeastern China and Tibet, northern India
- **Habitat:** Anywhere between the 42 north parallel and 33 south parallel.

Description: *Camellia sinensis* can grow up to 15 feet, but are pruned to 4-6 feet tall for tea production. The evergreen leaves are glossy, serrate, and elliptic. The white fragrant flowers become smooth, shiny capsules.

Gather together

Jessica Baker, LAc, RH (AHG)

History of Tea

There are numerous plants that arouse the urge for botanical piracy. *Camellia sinensis,* the plant that is called "cha," "te," and "tea" is one such plant. The Chinese knew how to grow, harvest and process the tea plant and controlled that information for centuries. Tea made its way to Europe from China around 1560. At first it was a drink for the aristocracy, but soon tea spread to the London coffee houses, where wealthy men gathered to conduct business. Britain's East India Company, in its ruthless quest for colonial control, was able to monopolize the tea trade by financing exports with illegal opium. This practice eventually led to China's military defeat and enforced trading agreements.

During this period, the East India Company smuggled plants and seeds from China and after many unsuccessful attempts, established Indian tea plantations in Assam and Sikkim. Tea was still virtually unknown in India until introduced by the British, although tea was one of the plants that traveled the Silk Road. The cultivation of tea in India led to drastic changes in trade and international politics, as it contributed to the perpetuation of Britain's colonial rule.

The demand for tea continued to rise in Europe as prices dropped enough for it to become a drink of the people, and not just the rich and aristocratic. People went to tea houses to catch up on local gossip and discuss politics. By 1750 in Britain, tea had surpassed ale and gin as the preferred drink of the lower class because of the taxes on alcohol. Charles II attempted to make the sale of tea in private houses forbidden—tea was taxed in liquid form, not dry—but it was impossible to enforce. Troubles with tea continued abroad, as well, as the demise of the British empire was partially due to loss of revenue from the colonies and the Boston Tea Party. With the duty tax on tea steadily rising, smuggling became profitable and tempting. Adulterating tea with other herbs like willow or licorice, and reusing dried tea became commonplace. Adulteration continued until the Food and Drug Act of 1875 threatened stiff penalties.

Elsewhere, tea was undergoing other transformations. It was in America in 1680 that the addition of milk was first mentioned. At the World Trade Fair of 1904, ice was first added to samples to entice drinkers on a hot day. Thomas Sullivan of New York developed tea bags when he realized one of his restaurant clients brewed his samples still in the wrapping to avoid the mess. The demand for sugar rose with the consumption of tea, as it was added for its caloric value, giving the drinker an instant energetic high.

Although tea is native to parts of India, the commercial cultivation of tea did not begin there until after the practice was introduced by the ruling British. Tea is now synonymous with India, as Darjeeling and Assam have become household names among tea drinkers. There are *chaiwallas*, or tea stands, all over India and Nepal. They are humble places that serve hundreds of cups of tea to all kinds of people. There are exotic stores that only sell the finest and rarest tea varieties. Chai is now popular in the West as well, the creamy spiced tea having warmed its way into people's hearts.

At the same time, our rituals around tea, long practiced in China, were developing around the world. Anna, 7th Duchess of Bedford, is credited with having started afternoon tea in the early 1800s. Dinner was generally not served until eight o'clock and the gap between lunch and dinner was too long to go without refreshments. Anna proposed tea and light snacks in the late afternoon, and the custom spread into wealthier homes, where servants would set the tables with silver tea sets, expensive china, and a plethora of sandwiches and scones and cream. High tea reached the working class, too. It was a time for people to gather and talk, and eat what would be the main meal for many. Afternoon or high tea continues to be a ritual in Britain, and beyond. It is an opportunity to drink tea, talk about home and work, and indulge in pastries and cream.

Southern Delicacy

Sweet tea still fuels the South. I have even heard it said that sweet tea has the South by the balls. I have to agree. Locals will tell you that you can't survive a summer in the South without sweet tea. All family, church and community functions are required to have sweet tea or no one will show up. At these functions I have heard many southern men say, "Honey, will you get me some more sweet tea?" their tones as noxiously sweet as the syrupy drink they are asking for. Men, women and children alike drink sweet tea by the Mason-jar full. I can attest there is nothing like a tall, cold glass of sweet tea on a sticky, hot southern afternoon.

Bittersweet Memories

My own memories of sweet tea are bittersweet. The drinking of tea happens within the home, but also revolves around the gathering of friends and family. As much as I loved congregating with my family, it also filled me with sadness. It was a reminder that I was different, isolated and detached.

Due to urinary tract issues and a ureter tube surgery at age nine, I was told I would need to stay away from caffeinated and alcoholic beverages. Being that young, this news didn't mean much since all I drank was milk, water, Kool-aid and unsweetened fruit juice anyway. As I got into my teenage years and my friends began to drink sweet tea, soda and alcohol, I began to occasionally drink with them as well. I grew to love sweet tea. The combination of bitter and sweet, congealed into a caramelized tea infusion, is oh so good.

The alkaloids in caffeine surging through my young veins, I felt energized from both tea and sugar, two things I didn't often consume. These binges did not serve me well and I continued to have urinary tract infections (UTIs) through my teenage years. UTIs meant antibiotics and antibiotics meant vaginal candidiasis, or yeast infections. The stress of having chronic inflammation and infections were exacerbated by my consumption of bread, alcohol and sugar. Unknowingly, I was feeding the continuous cycle of inflammation, infection and medication. My health made me feel even more separated from my friends and family, and was a constant distraction that other people my age didn't have to deal with.

I don't know how I would have reacted if the tea would have been warm and unsweetened instead of sweet and iced. In Chinese medicine, the combination of cold (iced) and damp (sugar) can lead to a lack of digestive fire, which is further aggravated by continuous antibiotic use. Antibiotics are also cold in nature and kill all bacteria in your body, even the beneficial gut flora needed to have a healthy digestive tract. I also had a diet heavy in processed food, bread and cheese. The combination of all these factors, along with my constitutional kidney deficiency, kept me susceptible to a cycle of imbalance.

By the time I moved to California at age twenty-one, I was completely out of balance from a lifetime of infections and antibiotic use. Lifestyle habits, family issues and poor nutrition had me anxious, fearful, defensive and irritable. Working with herbs and nutrition, it took years for me to bring myself into balance. The shift to health was necessary, as my anxiety, depression, and constant yeast infections left me feeling like I would never feel good again. After a lifetime of pretty continuous antibiotic use, it took seven years to eliminate the irritating substances from my life. Two years on a strict candida diet to eliminate all the yeast from my body was a life-saver. By the time I started my master's degree in traditional Chinese medicine in 2004, I had a deep connection with herbs, my health had greatly improved, and my entire outlook on life had changed. I still didn't drink much caffeinated tea, but that was about to change.

Mythical Beginnings

Being a student of Chinese medicine gave me a deep appreciation for *Camillia sinensis*. There is a legend of how tea came to use in China, in 2737 BC. Shen Nong, The Divine Farmer, who was the father of agriculture, herbalism and animal husbandry, was resting and was woken by the aroma coming from a pot of boiling water. The pot contained the fallen leaves of a nearby bush and he was enticed by the smell emanating from the steam. Shen Nong tasted the infusion and stated that it gave him "vigour of body, contentment of mind, and determination of purpose." By the Tang Dynasty (618-906 AD), "cha" was the name for tea, which consisted of fresh green leaves that had been picked, pressed into cakes, roasted to a reddish hue and boiled with a little salt. The bricks of tea were easily transported along the Silk Road to India and Turkey, and so the world's fascination with tea began.

Tea Ceremony

In 2008 I had the opportunity to study in Hangzhou, China, through a partnership between Five Branches University and Zhejiang University. While there, I went to the Long Jing tea plantation. Gazing upon acres of old tea terraces I could feel the intimate connection between the land and the people who had cultivated this plant since at least the 3rd century AD. I was transported back in time, when *Lu Cha, Camellia sinensis*, was an appreciated gift to the Chinese people. A nutritive tonic that reduces hunger, refreshes the mind, and relieves thirst and irritability; *Lu Cha* is the link to the survival and longevity of the Chinese people. Standing among the rows of plants, this connection is palpable. At Long Jing, the tea is still harvested and processed by hand. The love of the plant resonates with all who work there.

At Long Jing, we experienced a traditional tea ceremony. All tea comes from the same plant, *Camillia sinensis*. We were told the history of the plantation and how its farmers still practice agricultural techniques from a thousand years ago. We were given the first, second, and third harvests off a tea plant and encouraged to taste the difference in smell, taste, and bodily sensations. Each glass was poured with elegant consistency, as tea masters take their art seriously. After the ceremony we walked around the grounds, and I saw men heating leaves to halt the oxidation and ensure these leaves became green tea and not something darker. The rhythm of the cast-iron bowls was constant, worked by hands that look weathered from the heat of the metal. I gazed across the ponds at the rock sculptures and the turtles bathing in the sun. It seemed timeless. I thought of the relationship between man and tea, the ancient knowledge of tea preparation, which is rooted in reverence, observation, and curiosity.

I learned that white tea is made from the youngest shoots of the tea plant, hand-processed with no oxidation. They provide a subtle, sweet flavor. Green tea is made from leaves allowed to wither slightly before oxidation is stopped by rapidly heating the leaves. Green tea has a sweet earthy taste that can become bitter if steeped for more than a couple of minutes. Oolong tea comes from leaves that have been partially oxidized. Oolongs have a fragrant, intriguing taste and aroma. Black tea is made from leaves that have been fully oxidized, which gives the leaves the dark brown and black color. The flavors are more robust and the caffeine content is higher than in white, green, and oolong varieties. Puer is aged black tea, which was illegal to import into the United States until 1995. Puer has a strong earthly taste with a rich aroma. It was the earthy smell of puer that led to its ban in the US, as officials thought the tea had molded and wouldn't allow it to be transported into the country.

Chinese Medicine

Lu Cha is known to harmonize the stomach and relieve the nausea and vomiting that arise from rebellious stomach *Qi*. Damp accumulation in the intestines can also cause diarrhea and the bitter quality of *Lu Cha* dispels this dampness. An infusion of *Lu Cha* taken with food will reduce excess fat or oil and is often used for weight loss. Once again, the bitter quality disperses dampness and releases it through the intestines. For deficiency of the digestion, a soup of *Lu Cha* with onions and ginger can be taken daily. *Lu Cha* also clears the head and brings clarity of thought and mental acuity. It is the action of dispelling dampness that brings more *Qi* and blood flow to the brain. When there is more nourishment to the brain, mental alertness, creativity, intuition, and intellect are enhanced.

Research into cancer treatment is now demonstrating *Lu Cha's* properties of longevity. The antineoplastic and antimutagenic properties of *Camillia sinensis* are coming to light as polyphenols are studied for their cytoprotective effects and their ability to inhibit the carcinogenic byproducts of chemotherapy. Different metabolites in the fermentation of tea are demonstrating effects against chemical mutagens. Green tea is also reported to reverse MRSA and PRSA, the more difficult strains of *Staphylococcus* infections. We have only just begun to study the benefits of this plant with Western research techniques, but the intimate knowledge possessed by the ancient Chinese is well documented and worthy of our appreciation and respect.

Moderation is Key

Camillia sinensis is a central nervous system stimulant and may cause nervousness, rapid heartbeat, insomnia, increased blood glucose and cholesterol levels, and high levels of stomach acid. For those who have an overactive central nervous system, it would be best to minimize tea ingestion. People with stomach *Qi* deficiency who experience nausea when drinking green tea should drink processed tea, such as black tea or oolong, which are gentler on the stomach. The addition of honey and milk can also help reduce the unpleasant experiences.

As long as I am well rested and hydrated, I can drink tea almost daily. There are times I know I am drinking too much. As I write this, I should probably drink more herbal tea, instead of leaning on *Camilla* so heavily to be alert and focused. It is partially in the interest of science that I take it to the limit at times. Other times, it is my own journey of self-care and priorities that perpetuate my habit. My preference is now for hot tea—my personal favorites are French lavender Earl Grey and Darjeeling—but when I am in the South or it's a hot summer day and I get the craving for a glass or two of sweet tea, I will delightfully indulge.

My bittersweet relationship to tea has changed. Instead of the discomfort caused by caffeine and sugar, my body is strong enough to accept a little appeasement. I have entertained many friends with celebrations of afternoon tea. As long as I don't have more than a cup or two (or three), I feel awake and vibrant, connected to those with whom I am sharing the ancient tradition of storytelling, laughing, and drinking tea.

Tea's Song

Whether it's southerners on a Sunday, the British in the afternoon, or a Chinese tea ceremony, tea brings people together and has for thousands of years. The trade of tea altered the evolution of societies, economies, and cultures as this elusive plant captured hearts, minds and stomachs around the world. Tea reminds us that we all belong here, regardless of our differences. Tea reminds us that we are all family, connected by our presence on Earth.

Gather together

Tea Recipes

Southern Sweet Tea

Ingredients:
- 1 cup turbinado sugar ("Church sweet" is 1.5-2 cups.)
- 7 bags of orange pekoe tea
- 1 gallon of water

Boil 1 quart of water and remove from heat. Add tea bags to boiled water and steep for 7 minutes. Add sugar to hot water and mix well. Pour tea and remaining water into a glass gallon pitcher. Stir well. Fill a tall glass 3/4 full of ice and fill with tea. Gulp deeply.

Green Tea Face Mask

Ingredients:
- 1 ounce powdered green tea
- 1 ounce powdered rose buds
- 1 ounce powdered lavender flowers
- 1 ounce almond meal
- 3 ounces French green clay (or bentonite clay)

Mix all powdered herbs, almond meal and clay together. Keep the mixture in the refrigerator. For one mask, take out 1-2 tbsp. of the mixture and add enough honey to moisten. Apply to face, neck and décolletage. Let sit for 10-15 minutes, making sure the mask stays moist to avoid over-drying the skin. Gently remove mask with a warm cloth. After the mask, mist with hydrosol of your choice (I like rose) and moisturize.

Antioxidant Tisane

- 1 tsp. green tea
- 1 tsp. tulsi basil
- 1 slice of lemon

Steep green tea and tulsi basil in boiled water for 3-5 minutes. Strain out herbs. Squeeze in one slice of lemon and add honey if desired. Sip while tea is warm.

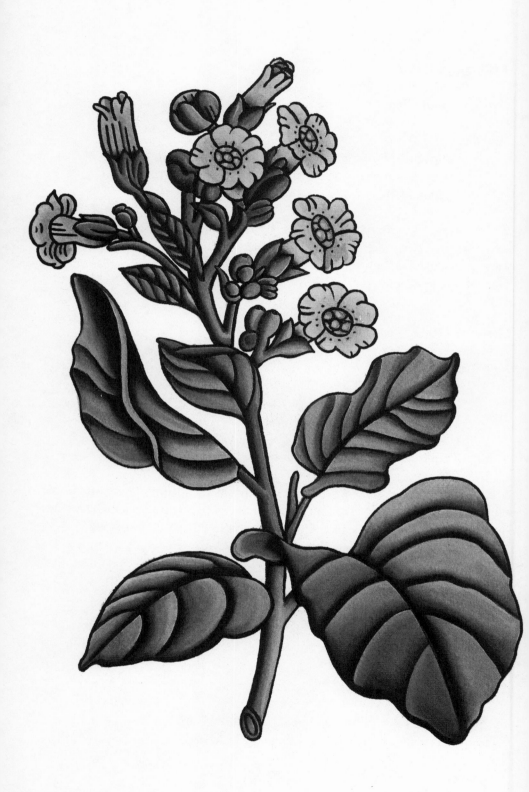

CHAPTER SEVEN

Tobacco: Connect With Spirit

Nicotiana rustica
- **Properties**: Spicy, Bitter, Warm
- **Meridians entered**: Lung, Large Intestine
- **Elements influenced**: Metal
- **Original habitat**: Andes region of South America

Nicotiana quadrivalvis
- **Properties**: Spicy, Bitter, Warm
- **Meridians entered**: Lung, Large Intestine
- **Elements influenced**: Metal
- **Original habitat**: West of the Rocky Mountains

Nicotiana tabacum
- **Properties**: Spicy, Bitter, Warm
- **Meridians entered**: Lung, Large Intestine
- **Elements influenced**: Metal
- **Habitats**: Cultivated in the southern US, China, Brazil, and India for commercial production.

Description: *Nicotiana* species are primarily annuals that can grow from 3-10 feet tall. The large alternate leaves are ovate to lanceolate, spiraling around the stem. The leaves are harvested for the tobacco industry so the fragrant tubular flowers are often cut before they bloom. The flowers range in color from white to cream, pink to red. The fruits are oval to elliptic capsules filled with numerous small brown seeds.

Connect with Spirit
Connect with Yourself

Ancestral Medicine

Oh tobacco, what a bad rap you have. And oh, how I love you in ways I'm not supposed to admit. Although I haven't smoked cigarettes in years I still smoke in my dreams, not every night or every other night, but sometimes. And when I wake in the morning I'm filled with a deep contentment I don't quite understand. The sacred tobacco that has been the material connection to Spirit for centuries in Native American cultures has become demonized, because the abuse and treatment of this plant has made it one of the world's most prolific killers. Tobacco played a constant role in my childhood and the aroma of burning tobacco evokes many memories of my past, of my relatives and my ancestors.

My memories of moving around as a child are ones of sadness, apprehension and fear. When I found out we would be moving from Texas to Germany, I was deeply upset that I would not be starting junior high with friends that I had known the last three years. I literally threw a temper tantrum at the age of twelve. I cried, screamed and kicked until my parents reminded me of my age and told me to stop. Ridiculous to me now, since moving to Europe as a teenager is one of the coolest things imaginable. But at the time it was just another loss. It was another realization that these friends would also slip into the past and become vague recollections of youth.

Moving to Germany would distance me even further from my extended family, whom I saw maybe only a few days every year or two. While in Germany, the smell of tobacco—daily in our house because my dad was a heavy smoker at the time—would sometimes evoke memories of my family back home. In my daydreams, I would yearn for closeness to them. I would think of my maternal great-grandmother, Irene, with her ornate snuff box, surrounded by all of her chain-smoking sisters and brothers. I'd think of my great aunts with their raspy voices, wrinkled skin, yellow stained teeth and fingers, most of them hardened, irritable women. They would sit at granny's table, inhale mouthfuls of smoke and coffee at the same time, and bitch about someone in the family. Some were playful and kind but it was hard to get past the smoke and judgments to get close enough to find out. My grandma Frances quit smoking cigarettes decades before her passing, but when I would visit, I loved watching her as she got ready for work. Her personal bathroom, a mixture of hairspray, tobacco smoke and perfume, was where she would perform her elaborate ritual of beautification. With a make-up brush in one hand and a cigarette in the other, she exuded beauty and strength. Like her, most of the women on my mom's side succumbed to smoking-related illnesses like lung cancer, emphysema, chronic obstructive pulmonary disease (COPD) and heart disease. The legacies of these women live on, even as my memories of them fade like the smoke that engulfed them.

When I went to see my grandma, it also meant time with my cousins. During my youth, all my cousins were girls except the youngest. They all lived within twenty minutes of grandma, and a couple of them were usually staying with her. When we were between the ages of about ten and sixteen, we cousins would gather in groups to take our "walk around the block," which meant walking grandma's neighborhood—about four square blocks—as an excuse for some of us to smoke cigarettes that had been stolen from some adult, hang out alone without supervision, meet up with boys, and generally explore the neighborhood. Although I had a few puffs of cigarettes here and there, I didn't start smoking regularly until I was seventeen.

Like many others, I started smoking cigarettes to self-medicate. I had smoked tobacco a few times in junior high, but it wasn't until my senior year in high school that I became a smoker. That year, the only high-school boyfriend I'd ever had cheated on me and I was devastated. My friends and family always told me cigarettes calmed their nerves and relaxed them, so I decided I wanted one. I was in the car with my cousin Aimee when I told her I wanted a cigarette. She said, "Really?" in that thick southern drawl she has. "Yes, really," I said, only saying it because I knew my ex hated smoking and I wanted to rebel against everything he stood for. She handed me a cigarette and lighter and looked at me as I put it to my lips and lit it. I inhaled deeply and choked. I took another hit, coughed a little, and then felt the tension in my shoulders relax. I sighed. I was hooked. I began to smoke every time I wanted to cry. Within a year I became a two-pack-a-day smoker and I began to experiment with cannabis, psilocybin and other mind- and mood-altering substances.

As I moved away from home for the University of Georgia, my cigarette smoking increased as I began to stress out about my parent's impending divorce and the disillusionment I felt towards life in general. I developed a nasty cough and got bronchitis several times my sophomore year in college. Finally the doctor at the student health clinic said, "Look, certain people can smoke for years without negative effects, but you can't. You have to quit." Of course I already knew that but I did wise up and I listened to him. By then I had done enough soul-searching to know that I had begun smoking cigarettes as a crutch, at first as a way to escape my emotions and later as a way to deal with the stress of graduating high school and moving off to college. Smoking was also a great socializing tool. I made many friends smoking cigarettes at clubs and outside of Reed Hall at UGA. I was in tune with myself enough to know the real reason I smoked.

Chinese Medicine

It wasn't that hard to stop smoking. Once I realized that I would have chronic bronchitis if I continued, I quit. It was a little hard when I was up late with friends, hanging out or studying, but overall I didn't crave nicotine much after the first couple of weeks. I could breathe so much better and I now noticed how the stench of cigarette smoke was leaving my clothes and bedroom. I also realized why I had started smoking in the first place. At that time, the grief over the betrayal of my boyfriend was overwhelming. I felt betrayed, embarrassed, and partially responsible for his actions. I wanted to punish myself for being vulnerable, for getting so intimately close to someone, for being so naive and stupid. One way I punished myself was to smoke cigarettes, something I knew was addictive and unhealthy. Now I no longer felt the need to punish myself and so I didn't.

I wasn't aware of it when I quit, but in Chinese medicine there is a connection between grief and the Lungs. We have a spiritual entity residing within us known as our *Po*. *Po* is thought of as our corporeal soul, a somatic expression of the human soul, that returns to the Earth when we die. *Po* is housed in the lungs and resides in specific areas in the body. When our *Shen Xian*, or eternal spirit, is content, our *Po* fills us with acceptance, love, and compassion. When it's out of balance, our *Po* is fueled by self-destructive thoughts and behavior. Our *Po* is sometimes called the seven stinking daggers. As in Jerry Alan Johnson's book on medical qi gong, they are the manifestations of negative thoughts and emotions, of hostility and aggression:

> *Fei Du*, or Flying Poison: arrogance and pride.
> *Chu Hui*, or Sprouting Filth: shame and guilt that lead to anxiety.
> *Fu Shi*, or Flying Arrow: hopelessness and ignorance.
> *Chou Fei*, or Stinking Lungs: greed and selfish desires.
> *Shi Kou*, or Corpse Dog: unresolved traumas, dwelling on the past.

Que Yin, or Yin Bird, also referred to as the "night tormentor": negative judgments, jealousy, resentment.

Tun Zei, or Sipping Thief: the feeling of never having enough, never being satisfied.

When we harbor negative feelings about others, and ourselves, we feed *Po*. Beating ourselves up for it only emboldens *Po* more. It's hard not to beat up on yourself, especially when so many people around us are beating themselves up too. It's why we have so many judgments of others. It is why we can be so violent with our words and our actions. We are a society full of people who don't really like themselves. We can no longer see the preciousness of our own existence. Because of that, we can't see the preciousness of anything else's existence. Our collective *Po* is out of control and we can't get out of the cycle. It's a hard cycle to break when our *Po* have gotten so strong from generations of the shame, guilt, and fear that have been perpetuated through religion and patriarchal society. To quell the overactive *Po*, we must be able to access the high vibrations of the *Dao* through our *Shen Xian*, or eternal spirit. Tobacco has often been used a method for this.

Sacred Medicine

As humans we have a long history of tobacco use. Instead of cursing our addiction to it, let us remember that tobacco is sacred to millions of people, and has been for thousands of years. *Nicotiana rustica* has been cultivated in the Andes Mountains for about seven thousand years, where various tribes have used it to access the wisdom of the universe and deepen their connections to spirit. By the time the Spanish invaders came, tobacco was being cultivated from Chile to Quebec.

Many people use tobacco in ritual and daily life with different customs surrounding its use. For many native people, tobacco is one of the four sacred plants, held in reverence with its three sisters: maize, squash and beans. Table 1 shows how widespread tobacco and its various uses are in South America.

Table 1—Traditional tobacco use in South America

Rolled and inhaled through nostrils	233 tribes
Inhaled as snuff	53 tribes
Licked	16 tribes
Drank as an infusion	64 tribes
Chewed	56 tribes
Eaten as food	15 tribes

In many South American tribes, tobacco is thought to be one of many visionary hallucinogenic plants. The Shipibo-Conibo distinguish between two kinds of religious practitioners: the seers who uses tobacco, and the *ayahuasqueros* who use *Banisteriopsis caapi* combined with other psychotropic plants, including tobacco. Both the seer and the *ayahuasquero* gain transcendental, complex images that give insight into the unique way they observe the world. These images can be seen in the elaborately beautiful textiles woven by Shipibo-Conibo women.

Dale Pendell writes in *Pharmakopeoia*, "Tobacco provides what every shaman must undergo: sickness, death, and rebirth." The dreams and visions the tobacco seer has during his catatonic state bring back messages from the spirit world. Tobacco also grows prolifically on gravesites throughout South America. This was not unnoticed by the native people, and the offering of tobacco began as a way to communicate with ancestors and spirits. The Mundurucú believe that the first tobacco plant grew where the tobacco-spirit was buried, when still in human form. Yaruro shamans blow smoke over hunters, fishermen, and gatherers to protect them from danger and guarantee an abundance of food. At least as early as 1500 BC, Mayans were smoking tobacco ceremoniously prior to battles, hunting expeditions, and for rituals of fertility. Throughout many cultures, smoke links the human world to the spirit world and is an offering to the creator for giving and sustaining life.

Commercialization of the Sacred

As the colonizers began to cultivate *Nicotiana tabacum* and send it back to Europe, the aristocratic hunger for this new exotic plant spread through the continent. Tobacco was the new panacea, sold by physicians to cure anything.

To understand the value of tobacco at this time, you must know that tobacco was a form of currency for over two hundred years. The commercial success of tobacco fueled the slave trade, as 13% of the colonies' population was slaves. The cultivation of tobacco, like all crops, relied heavily on slave labor. The wealth provided by tobacco was the catalyst for the end of British rule in the New World, as colonial financial independence became possible.

The Poison Path

Unlike the native tobacco smoked among the colonizers and the tribes of South America, cigarettes today contain more than 600 ingredients. Even without the added chemicals, it is no surprise tobacco was embraced by the masses in Europe and North America. Tobacco contains the para-sympathomimetic alkaloid nicotine. In its free form, nicotine is highly fat-soluble and is absorbed by all tissues of the body. In the GI tract it is absorbed 100%, which is why enemas of tobacco and ginger have been used for helminthic infestation. Nicotine is metabolized rapidly and is removed from the body during urination, so repeated inhalation or use is required to maintain nicotine levels in the body. Nicotine molecules are similar to acetylcholine and will bind to cholinergic receptors to give a stimulatory (in small doses) or a depressant (in large doses) effect. Nicotine has been used to enhance cognition, focus and alertness.

Indole alkaloids are also present in tobacco, and can affect mood and behavior by increasing serotonin levels and inhibiting monoamine oxidase. In high doses, ingestion of these alkaloids can cause visual hallucinations, dilated pupils, sweating and nausea. The hallucinatory action is not known but it is theorized that it could be similar to the action of LSD, which temporarily binds to serotonin receptors. Indole alkaloids are found in other hallucinogenic plants like *Banisteriopsis caapi,* the vine necessary for the ceremonial brew ayahuasca. It may be the physiological effect of these molecules that make both ayahuasca and tobacco so revered by humanity.

Tobacco's Song

My own use of tobacco was not hallucinogenic, but I did smoke countless cigarettes with friends while hanging out late into the night, sometimes on psychedelics. With each inhalation, I breathed in the intimacy of our shared experience. With each exhalation, we vocalized our hopes and fears, musing on life, death, and the future. These exchanges into the early hours of the morning happened in the presence of Spirit, whether we were aware of it or not. It was in sharing these moments and stories that my adulthood began to take form.

Connect with Spirit
Connect with Yourself

Tobacco Recipes

Spirit Offering

Sit quietly in front of a tree or plant that you find yourself drawn to. With an open heart and mind, give an offering of tobacco to the plant. As you tune into its vibration, feel the presence of its being and listen to any messages it wishes to share.

Herbal Smoking Blend

1 ounce each of the following dried herbs, roughly ground:
- Plantain leaves
- Yerba santa

1/2 ounce each of the following dried herbs, roughly ground:
- Mullein leaf
- Spearmint
- White Sage

1/4 ounce each of the following dried herbs, roughly ground:
- Lobelia leaf
- Violet leaf

A pinch of tobacco and/or cannabis.

Mix all herbs together and keep in a glass or metal container. Roll "joints" as needed to smoke or burn for contemplation, celebration or ritual. This is a good recipe to use when one is trying to stop smoking tobacco. It can be blended alone or with a small amount of tobacco or cannabis to enhance psychoactive properties.

Smoker's Support Tincture

- 1 ounce fresh dandelion root
- 1 ounce fresh marshmallow root
- 1 ounce fresh yellow dock root
- 1/2 ounce fresh mullein root and leaf
- 1/4 ounce fresh violet leaf
- 1/8 ounce fresh lobelia leaf
- 8 ounces high-proof alcohol

If you have a grinder or blender strong enough for roots; grind roots, plant material, and alcohol together until it is a thick mush. If not, cut roots and leaves as small as possible and add to alcohol. Put mixture in a glass jar with lid and sit in a cool dark location for one month, shaking daily. Always label and date! Strain out herbs after one month. Bottle tincture and take 5-10 drops each day to clear heat from the lungs and tissues.

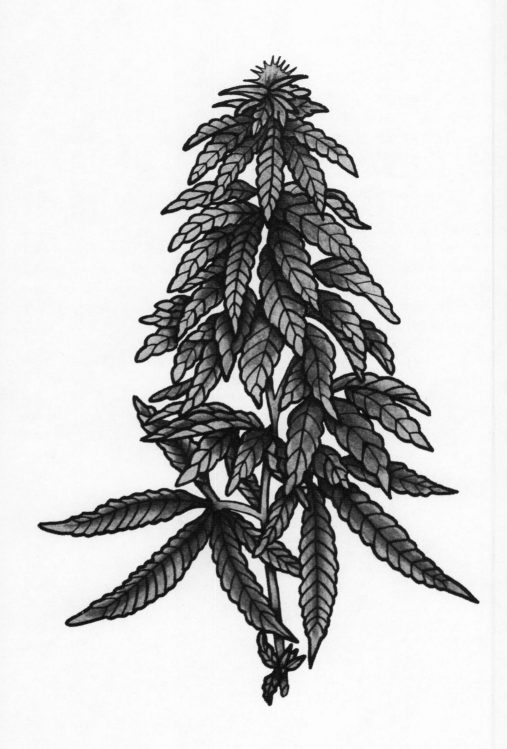

CHAPTER EIGHT

Cannabis: Reflect, Feel, Create, Evolve

Cannabis sativa
Marijuana, Ganja, Weed
Huo Ma (Ren)

- **Properties (of seeds)**: Sweet, Neutral
- **Meridians entered**: Large Intestine, Spleen, Stomach
- **Elements influenced**: Metal, Earth
- **Original habitat**: May have originated in Central Asia, found in the northwest regions of the Himalayas, throughout China and western Asia—Iran to India.
- **Habitats**: Fluvial deposits on crags and stony slopes; nitrogen-rich soils near human habitations; cultivated across the world in a variety of conditions.

Description: Cannabis plants are primarily annual, although they are perennial in temperate locations. Cannabis can grow up to 20 feet tall with extensive branching. They are dioecious, having with only one sex on an individual plant, although both male and female flowers can occur on a single plant. Both male and female plants are needed to produce seeds. The leaves are palmately compound with serrate leaflets. The flowers on female plants, called buds, are dense, elongate clusters that grow on the pistillate. The buds are various shapes of green with white that turns to orange or red. The flowers are what is harvested for recreational and medicinal use. The male flowers grow in clusters and produce pollen that fertilizes the buds. The seeds are oblong and various shades of brown.

Reflect
Feel
Create
Evolve

Evolution

Cannabis is one of the plants that illuminate me to the infinite possibilities of life. The entire cannabis plant embodies the versatility we are all capable of. For centuries the hemp stalk has been used for fiber and fuel, the seed for food and medicine, the flowers and resins for enlightenment and recreation. Hemp cord identified in pottery dating from over 10,000 years ago has been found in Taiwan. In 2009, Richard Hamilton wrote an article on sustainable agriculture for *Scientific American*, pointing out that this use of hemp coincided with the dawn of agriculture. He writes, "Modern humans emerged some 250,000 years ago, yet agriculture is a fairly recent invention, only about 10,000 years old... Agriculture is not natural; it is a human invention. It is also the basis of modern civilization." In *Dragons of Eden: Speculations on the Origin of Human Intelligence*, Carl Sagan postulates that "...in human history the cultivation of marijuana led generally to the invention of agriculture, and thereby to civilization." Botanist Li Hui-Lin wrote that in China, "...the use of Cannabis in medicine was probably a very early development. Since ancient humans used hemp seed as food, it was quite natural for them to also discover the medicinal properties of the plant." Cannabis has been mentioned in classical Chinese texts dating as far back as 2800 BC, when it is written that Emperor Shen Nong taught the people how to cultivate "*Ma*" (hemp) for making cloth. Around 200 AD, Hua Tou, a famous Chinese physician, used cannabis as an anesthetic during surgery. In 1578, Li Shih-Chen wrote of the antibiotic and antiemetic effects of cannabis. Modern Chinese herbal medicine books such as *Chinese Medical Herbology and Pharmacology*, by John Chen and Tina Chen, list cannabis seeds (*Huo Ma Ren*) as a valuable medicine to lubricate the intestines, nourish yin and clear heat.

Endocannabinoid System

The latest research by the scientists at Phytecs, a research group that develops and derives products from natural and synthetic sources that support and restore optimal endocannabinoid system function, is revealing that our endocannabinoid system (ECS) regulates almost every aspect of our physiology. In essence, there is a co-evolution of humans and cannabis, with results we are only beginning to comprehend.

Human evolution with cannabis and other plant life is evident in our ECS and liver detoxification enzymes. Our ECS is a homeostatic regulatory system that is found throughout the body, in the brain, heart, bone, adipose tissue and organs. The ECS regulates mitochondrial activity, provides antioxidant protection and is responsible for the growth of and development of our nervous system. It also regulates mood, memory, appetite, pain levels and reward. Thanks to the work of Ethan Russo and other researchers we now know there are large concentrations of cannabinoid receptors in the skin, limbic system, cerebral cortex and cerebellum.

Many plants contain phytocannabinoids that bind to our endocannabinoids and have varied effects, like the reduction of inflammation and bactericidal properties. Cannabidiol (CBD) is the most common phytocannabinoid in fiber plants and is the second most prevalent in "marijuana" or "drug" cultivars. In studies performed in 2007 CBD was found to protect the brain from traumatic injury. CBD was also found to be more potent than ascorbate (Vitamin C) and tocopherol (Vitamin E) as an antioxidant. The United States government even has a patent on the neuroprotective activity of CBD. This means that US government understands the potential of cannabinoids as a way to prevent or stop the spread of nerve cell damage. This is significant in stroke, traumatic brain injury, and other head injuries. So if the government has a patent on CBD, then how can it continue to classify cannabis as a Schedule 1 drug, defining it as a plant that has no medicinal value whatsoever?

Other cannabinoids (CBG, CBC, CBT) have also been found in other plants, like rhododendron, liverwort and woody umbrella. Beta-caryophyllene is a cannabinoid present in virtually all plants, with high concentrations in cannabis. It is found to be anti-inflammatory and protective for gastric cells. Identifying cannabinoids in other plants helps us understand that cannabis is a medicinal herb, just like the countless other medicinal herbs we rely on. We see this directly when we witness cannabis's ability to reduce vomiting and nausea.

Anandamide is an endocannabinoid that is commonly called the "bliss molecule" because its activation elicits a relaxed, joyful response. Anandamide is also important for motor control, memory and higher thought processes. Acupuncture increases anandamide levels on the skin where needles are inserted. CB2 receptors are found throughout the skin and are activated with the stimulation of acupuncture needles. This could be the reason clients report feeling "high," relaxed, and spaced out during and after acupuncture sessions.

Aromatherapists have long known about the largest group of plant chemicals, terpenoids. Terpenoids, not cannabinoids—as most consumers think—are responsible for the aroma of cannabis. Terpenoids occur in complex and variable mixtures with marked structural diversity that seem to serve various ecological roles, like defense against pests and fungi (E. Russo, Taming THC: Potential Cannabis Synergy and Phytocannabinoid-Terpenoid Entourage Effect; British Journal of Pharmacology, 2011). Although there is much to be learned about the processes of the brain, we have substantial knowledge on the functions and purpose of the limbic system.

CB1 (cannabinoid 1) receptors are found in high concentrations throughout the brain, including within the limbic system. The limbic system, also called the primitive brain, plays an important role in arousal, memory, feeding, sexual behaviors and motivation. The limbic system controls olfaction (sense of smell) and is essential for the detection of toxic airborne molecules, predators, fires, and other dangers.

More research is needed as cannabis continues to gain traction as a powerful medicine for life-debilitating illnesses. Our endocannabinoid system, our long history of cultivation of cannabis, and written texts documenting cannabis as a medicinal plant more than 2,000 years ago make it evident that human health can greatly improve with the use of this plant. For the longevity and happiness of our species, the acceptance and understanding of cannabis is necessary. I am positive that we will continue our co-evolution with this remarkable plant.

Understanding Synergy

Due to prohibition, cannabis has been bred to have higher and higher amounts of THC, with little attention to the cannabinoids, terpenoids or other components of the plant. Just like with other illegal substances, prohibition has led to the manufacture of concentrated cannabis that is extremely strong and often dangerously made. In our attempts to isolate THC and other constituents we have lost the essential benefit of whole-plant medicine.

There is a synergistic effect to the combination of constituents in every plant. In cannabis, CBD may delay the onset of THC and help reduce the unwanted side effects of anxiety, heart palpitations and paranoia that can ensue for many consumers. I think the ongoing legalization of cannabis is going to deter some of these side effects, but even so, the combined effect of these constituents requires further study. We must remember the synergy of all chemical constituents as cannabis gains popularity as a medicinal herb. It is the whole plant medicine, not isolation of compounds, like CBD, that will prove the most healing.

Cannabis Culture

I personally love that heart-pounding, mind-racing high that smoking cannabis flowers elicits. That is when creativity and motivation strike and bring me deeper insight into my relationship with the cosmos. Some consumers get lost in the chaos of euphoria and are unable to integrate the insights cannabis provides. Instead of a feeling of oneness, where they tap into the universal energy and creativity, they have a feeling of isolation and introversion, and their senses become dulled. This can be situational or strain specific, but it can also be a reflection of where the person is in their healing process. Cannabis can highlight insecurities, doubts and fears, causing anxiety, fear and disorientation rather than healing. A lot of times these negative feelings bring awareness that leads to deeper healing. Cannabis is bringing to light issues the person has suppressed, either mentally or spiritually. Without a doubt, the medicinal and spiritual qualities of cannabis far outweigh the subjective negative effects.

The legalization of cannabis and its acceptance in the medical community is long overdue. I get giddy every time I see a cannabis dispensary. It brings back the fondest memories of standing in the middle of a ganja garden, feeling the warm Northern California breeze, smoking a joint, pruning the plants while listening to my solar-powered radio. This was the late 90's, and although growing medical cannabis was legal under California law, there was still eradication under CAMP (Campaign Against Marijuana Planting). The fear of imprisonment was real. Growing medicinal cannabis was not respected as it is now and people risked everything for their right to cultivate. There is something exhilarating and empowering about growing your own medicine. It makes me feel alive and connected to all the people who have cultivated cannabis over the ages. For those in Northern California that grew under fear of harassment and arrest, the legalization of medicinal and adult-use cannabis has the potential to change not only the lives of patients, but also cannabis growers. A lot of healing can occur when prohibition goes away. Like many, there are days when I still pine for the good old days, when cannabis growers were the freedom fighters, providing clandestine medicine to those in need.

Today, cannabis is highly regulated, packaged for consumers, in child-proof packaging, and probably contains ingredients like propylene glycol, butane residue, and/or refined sugar. Yum! Almost makes me want to go back to the outlaw days. Almost. The fear that cannabis prohibition perpetuates is something that I have trouble comprehending. The losses of community, family and character that have come from imprisoning nonviolent drug dealers and cannabis users far outweighs the negative effects cannabis can have on a person's health or psyche. As our culture evolves, we have to look at the bigger picture. Which is worse: ingestion of a safe plant for recreational purposes or knowingly ruining someone's life because they are growing an herb? It is an obvious choice if we care about people at all.

Irie Meditation

My relationship with cannabis is one of deep respect and love. My twenty years working with medical cannabis have given me the opportunity to explore the healing powers of this herb for myself. Through irie meditation I have gotten to know myself. I learned how to meditate, commune with nature, and understand my role in this lifetime. Cannabis has shown me how to step back and see what is important to me. There have also been times when I used cannabis to disconnect, to serve as a buffer from the harshness of our world. Cannabis, like anything, can be used to escape if that is your intention at the time.

Cannabis is a gift that helps to expand our minds to the infinite possibilities of evolution. This is evident in its role in the progression of human civilization. It is time to honor cannabis again for the medicine that it is. As we see a paradigm shift in the acceptance of cannabis I believe we will also notice a change in the consciousness of those who use it recreationally. I look forward to the day when we employ cannabis for the myriad uses it evolved to provide—for fiber, fuel, food, medicine and cultural enlightenment.

Cannabis's Song

My meditations with cannabis have brought insights into my soul that continue to shape who I am. Cannabis inspires you to live up to your true potential, to look beyond the accepted norm and become much more than you ever imagined. There is no limit to the greatness you can achieve.

> ***Reflect***
> ***Feel***
> ***Create***
> ***Evolve***

Cannabis Recipes

Cannabis Chai Tea

Ingredients:

- 3 grams dried cannabis flowers
- 1 tablespoon Assam or Darjeeling
- 1 crushed cardamom pod
- 1 inch piece of fresh ginger root
- 1/4 teaspoon fennel seeds
- 1/4 teaspoon dried orange peel
- teaspoon cinnamon powder

Simmer 4 ounces water, 4 ounces of milk (the fattier the better—whole milk or coconut milk), and all ingredients together for 20 minutes. Strain out cannabis and other ingredients and set aside. Drink 2-4 ounces of the tea as needed to promote appetite, reduce nausea or as a gentle relaxer.

Potent Protein Powder

Grind 1 pound of hemp seeds. Daily add 1 tbsp. to granola, yogurt or smoothie to boost your intake of essential fatty acids. Keep rest of the ground seeds in the refrigerator to prevent rancidity.

Keep It Regulated (Constipation Tea)

- 3-6 grams *Huo Ma Ren* (hemp seeds)
- 2-3 grams *Xing Ren* (apricot kernel)
- 3-6 grams *Shao Yao* (wild yam root)
- 2-3 grams *Zhi Shi* (immature bitter orange)
- 3-4 grams *Hou Po* (magnolia bark)
- 1-3 grams *Da Huang* (rhubarb rhizome and root - can be a strong purgative)
- This is a traditional Chinese formula for constipation due to dryness. Add all ingredients to a pint of water. Simmer herbs for 15-20 minutes. Strain herbs and set aside to be used in a second brewing of tea. Drink 4 ounces as needed to lubricate the bowels and promote bowel movement.

PART III

Young Adulthood/Awakeners

Psilocybin, Redwood, Yarrow, Nettle

Once I left Athens, Georgia and moved to Humboldt County, California I began to study herbalism, meditation, and other healing modalities. I was able to begin to heal from all the childhood traumas I experienced from illness and a life of moving around. For the first time, I felt I had a connection to the Earth, to plants, and most importantly, to myself. My study of herbalism awakened me to an innate understanding of our connection to our planet.

In Part III, I chose Psilocybin, for helping me see; Redwood, for nourishing me deeply; Yarrow, for awakening my spirit; and Nettle, for making me pay attention.

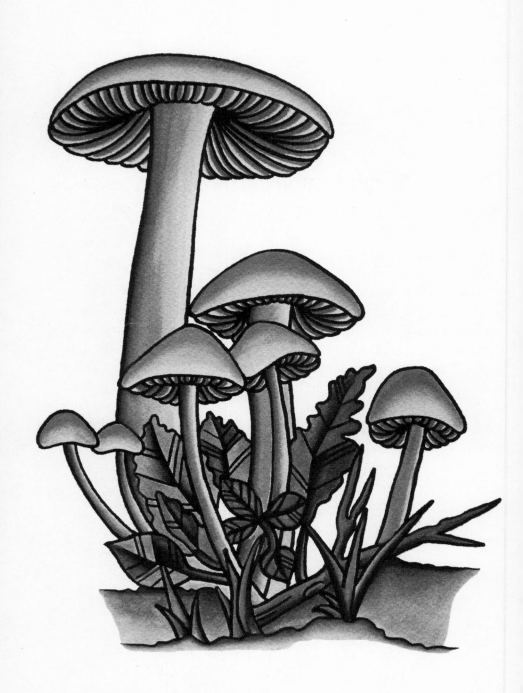

CHAPTER NINE

Psilocybin: See Yourself

Magic Mushrooms
Psilocybin cubensis

- **Properties:** Sweet, Bland, Cool
- **Meridians entered:** Stomach, Large Intestine, Liver, Heart
- **Elements influenced:** Earth, Metal, Fire
- **Original habitat:** humid grasslands in tropical and subtropical locations
- **Habitats:** Pastures where there is cow dung or moist dank locations.

Description: Psilocybin species vary in size and color but one distinguishing factor is the blue stain that occurs when the stalk is bruised. A spore print of the mushroom will be dark blue or dark purple. Always know proper identification of any mushroom before harvesting.

See yourself
Remember who you are

Spiritual Evolution

Psilocybin mushrooms like to fuck with me. Even before they have made it through my digestive system, they beckon me to take more. So sometimes I do, only to remember I should've waited for the first tasting to kick in. The cycle continues, and each time I remember I should have waited to see how strong they would be. At some point I tell myself not to listen to them and that I don't have to take more. Little tricksters they are, having integrated into our lives and culture millennia ago, transforming our language, culture, and spirituality each step of the way.

Co-evolution

Migration and mushrooms go hand-in-hand. Psychonaut and ethnobotanist Terence McKenna believes that psilocybin played a significant role in the evolution from *Homo erectus* to *Homo sapiens*. He theorizes that with the decrease of food supply, hunter-gatherers started following large herds of wild cattle and began eating the psilocybin that grew out of the dung. Small doses of this mushroom could have heightened their visual acuity and acted as a catalyst for abstract thought, religion, science, and philosophy. R. Gordon Wassen suggests hallucinogenic mushrooms are the causal agent for the appearance of spiritually aware human begins.

There are images of psilocybin mushrooms as spiritual substances dating back to the Cattle Cult and Cult of the Great Goddess from 9000 BC in Southern Anatolia. The Minoans, who have their roots in Egypt and Mesopotamia, used mushrooms in their spiritual practices. The most well-known mushroom cults are the Elysian Mysteries, the elusive rituals performed for the Goddess Demeter. Stones carved in the shape of mushrooms, dating between 500 BC and 900 AD, have been found in Guatemala, Mexico, Honduras and El Salvador. We indeed have a long history of using mushrooms for spiritual enlightenment.

I know that when I eat psilocybin or drink mushroom tea, I have an uncontrollable urge to commune with nature. My preference is to take a long walk through a redwood forest. The moistness among the redwood trees exudes life. I can breathe better, and I can feel the trees' vitality pulsating through my neural network. When on mushrooms, it's easier to notice that the trees and I breathe together, their exhale to my inhale, moving through this life together, as mycelium aids the trees roots in receiving life. Breathing as one.

Cosmic Connections

Mycelium is an organism made of countless hyphae (branching filaments) that create an intricate web of neural networking that mycologists call "the neurological network of nature." According to McKenna, mycelium traveled to our planet from outer space, along with other particles of cosmic energy that landed here in the distant past. It is known that it is the essential building block of soil and is the largest organism on Earth. Unlike plants, fungi and humans are heterotrophic and their dependence on organic matter has developed into complex cellular intelligence. The neural communication system allows for mycelium to spread for hundreds of miles and interact with countless other organisms. As mycologist Paul Stamets says, "The mycelial archetype can be seen throughout the universe in the formation of the Internet and in string theory." Mycelium is everywhere. And it needs to be for the reparation of the planet.

Mushroom Research

There is extensive research on mushrooms for bioremediation, toxic waste cleanup, and even for use as insecticide. Research performed by Paul Stamets on mycelium and medicinal mushrooms, including psilocybin, have revolutionized how we can work with mushrooms for everything from preventing colony death in beehives to specifically targeted insecticide that only kills a specific insect.

The prohibition of psilocybin has stifled the overwhelmingly beneficial effects of hallucinogenic mushrooms on physical and mental health and well-being. In the 1950s and 1960s there were over a thousand research papers written about LSD, psilocybin, and other psychedelic substances. Psychedelic-assisted psychotherapy was found to be more effective in treating alcoholism than current treatments, including AA. Recent studies on brain function on psilocybin show that psilocybin decreases ACC and mPFC activity, which are associated with anxiety and pessimism. In terminally ill cancer patients, a single dose of psilocybin, in conjunction with psychotherapy, led to a remarkable decrease in anxiety and depression compared to those given a placebo.

Mushroom Visions

My own experiences with psilocybin have given me a more optimistic, expanded life view. One of those experiences was on Mayan New Year, 2012. I had the most amazing life-affirming vision while on psilocybin. It was the end of a 52,000-year era and the beginning of another. The sun was rising over the jungle as I climbed to the top of Nohoc Mul, the tallest pyramid in the Yucatan, in Coba, with my husband and several friends. With each step, I knew we had climbed these steps together, countless times before. At the top, I gazed out of the small temple building and watched the sun shadow the landscape and the goddess temple. As the sun began to illuminate Xaibe, a rounded building thought to be an astronomical observatory, the memory began. It started with a beat, the heartbeat of the universe inside me, pulsating within me. As I looked out toward the observatory, I was in complete rhythm with it and the entire cosmos. I knew that I had been in this spot, thousands of years before. 52,000 years before, to be exact. I was there at the dawn of the last era as a medicine woman, a bridge between earth and the cosmos. I began to rock with the rhythm of the universe and then looked over and saw my friends as they once were and as they are today. My husband had a camera and said he wanted to document this occasion for all time. I knew he was the timekeeper, one who had documented important historical and astrological events thousands of years ago. I looked behind me and my friend Willow was speaking to a Japanese woman who had climbed Nohoc Mul to burn the incense of world peace, precisely at that moment. As they exchanged stories of where they were from I knew that their meeting was a continuation of our global migration and the importance of us all coming together and recognizing each other as one. As Willow handed me the incense, I burst into tears of joy and said, "Of course it's you, you have always been here and so have I." Slowly I came back into the present time and saw the entire progression and decline of Mayan civilization. I had been there, through it all.

Psilocybin and Our Psyche

Some say tripping on mushrooms is not a "real" experience. I am here to tell you that all experiences we have are real. Our reality is shaped by our culture, by the food we eat, the liquor that we drink, and the substances we take. It has always been that way. The difference today is that mind-altering pharmaceutical drugs are doing real damage to people's psyches.

We are flooded with anti-depressants, anxiolytics, mood stabilizers, benzodiazepines, and other psychoactive pharmaceuticals, and doctors are prescribing these without psychiatric supervision to such an extent that it borders on criminal. These pharmaceuticals are dangerous and without proper use can cause life-threatening conditions like serotonin syndrome. The side effects of these drugs can also include homicidal and suicidal thoughts. As we know, thoughts can lead to action. Have we looked into the connection between these drugs and the increase in mass shootings over the last ten years?

Research conducted since the 1950s has shown that psilocybin treats depression. Yet the medical establishment and the pharmaceutical industries would rather lobby to keep plant medicine illegal and knowingly harm the entire human population. There are many reasons for this. One of the more important reasons is that ingesting these mind-altering plants reminds us that we are one with all life on Earth. It awakens us to the fact that Mother Nature is our home, not our condo on the slopes or the lake house. With this knowing, we can change back into sentient, compassionate beings and not consumer-driven maniacs who are killing themselves while enriching corporations.

Psilocybin's Song

All mushrooms shift our consciousness and our patterns of behavior. As we connect to the web of life that mycelium encompasses, we remember that we are deeply connected to each other, to the planet, and to the cosmos. Then we find ourselves.

See yourself
Remember who you are

Psilocybin Recipes

Psilocybin Tea

- 1/8 ounce psilocybin mushrooms
- 3-inch slice of fresh ginger
- 2-4 cups water (depending on how strong you want tea)

Decoct mushrooms and ginger for 30 minutes, keep covered. Strain out mushrooms and keep liquid portion. Drink 1/2 cup of tea slowly. Wait for insights to appear.

Ooey Gooey Mushroom Honey

Fill a glass pint jar 1/2 full of dried psilocybin mushrooms. Fill same pint jar with honey. Let sit for 2-4 weeks. Strain out mushrooms and keep honey. Add a spoonful of honey to psilocybin tea or hot water.

Clear Sight Capsules

Powder 1 ounce dried psilocybin and 1 ounce dried reishi mushrooms together. Fill "00" caps with mushroom mixture. Take 1-2 capsules to help with clarity on a difficult situation.

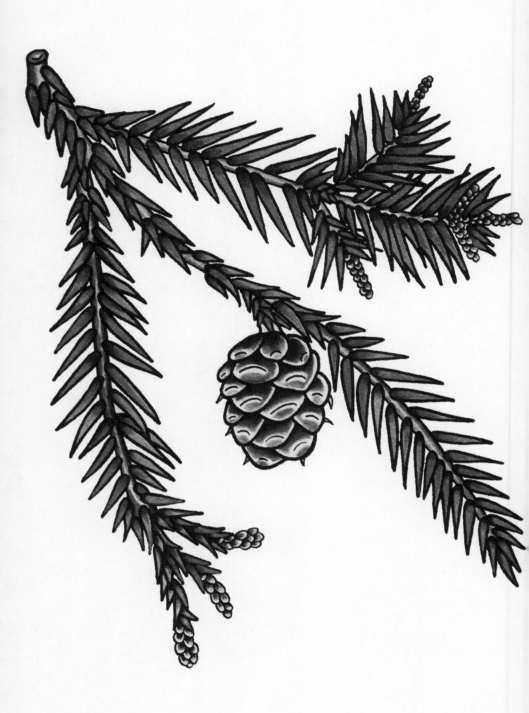

CHAPTER TEN

Redwood: Think Back, Slow Down, Listen, Remember

Sequoia sempervirens
Coast redwood

- **Properties**: Spicy, Sweet, Slightly Warm
- **Meridians entered**: Lung, Heart, Kidney
- **Elements influenced**: Metal, Fire, Water
- **Original habitat**: Coastal, central California to BC; relatives of the coastal redwood were present in the area 20 million years ago.
- **Habitats**: Coastal, Central California to BC.

Description: Redwood trees can grow over three hundred feet tall and live to be several thousand years old. The bark is red-brown, thick and fibrous with furrowed ridges. The leaves are alternate and have stomates on both surfaces. The adult leaves are flattened and linear or linear-lanceolate to deltate. The small, elliptical, reddish-brown female cones mature in one season.

Think Back
Slow Down
Listen
Remember

Evolution

In evolutionary terms, modern humans haven't been on the planet for very long. Our 200 years of industrialization, compared to the 144 million years for our modern *Sequoia*, would be almost insignificant if it weren't for the widespread death and destruction we have left in our wake. These gentle giants still remember what it was like when their relatives covered continents and housed countless species, from those high atop the ground in the redwood canopy down to the mycorrhiza attached to the roots in the soil. An ancient redwood forest houses over 350 vertical feet and millions of acres of diverse ecosystems, intact and essential to the survival of all life on Earth. Trees in the genus *Sequoia* were once present on three continents. Now they are reduced to a single species, *sempervirens* (the giant Sequoia is the genus *Sequoiadendron*), growing naturally only on the coast of California and Oregon. On public lands we only have around 81,500 acres of old-growth and second-growth coastal redwood forests. This is less than 5% of their original extent. In the United States we only have 2% of our forested land left. We are only beginning to see the ramifications of clear-cut logging operations.

Tree Time

In Humboldt County I saw firsthand what unsustainable logging practices do to the biodiversity of an ancient forest. I also saw how community activism could bring international attention to the devastation of an ancient ecosystem.

In 1997, I had just dropped out of college and was searching for some deeper meaning to my life. I was studying Greek and classical literature at the University of Georgia, while reading books on Daoism, yoga, quantum physics, and anything metaphysical I could get my hands on. I yearned to feel connected to something, yet felt incredibly uncomfortable in my own body. Even in my head, where I have always been sharp, I felt uneasy and conflicted. So much societal programming was being erased, as the wisdom I was gaining from my intellectual and spiritual studies began to rewire patterns that were older than my ancestors. The mystical experiences I was having with meditation and with psychedelic and psychotropic substances were opening me to dimensions I had only read about, but there was still something missing. I knew there was more and I knew I would find it if I kept searching.

That summer I moved to Fieldbrook, California with my boyfriend, who is now my husband. When we arrived, we did not want a television so we spent most of our time listening to local radio stations. Our favorite was KMUD, a local station centered on community activism in southern Humboldt County. By the mid-nineties, the fight between Pacific Lumber (Maxxam Corporation) and environmental activists was at a high point. When I got there in August 1997, local activist and musician Judi Bari had recently passed away and there was a collective sense that we had to save what was left of our forests and beat the evil corporations for Judi, for the salmon, for all species on Earth. KMUD had constant updates on where illegal logging was happening and where activists should meet for blockades and protests. We began going to rallies and getting involved in the movement. We provided company, food and supplies to an activist sitting in a tree called Mariah and we witnessed the violence he and other activists suffered at the hands of those who believed the propaganda perpetuated by the Maxxam Corporation. Mariah was eventually saved from logging but unfortunately, 73% of the Freshwater Watershed was logged, along with millions of acres of old-growth forests in the Pacific Northwest.

My time in the redwoods made me aware of a depth of beauty that cannot be described unless experienced and gave me a deeper purpose, a calling, a voice. I know that the redwood trees brought me back to life. When I landed in Humboldt, I felt like a shell of myself. My parents were getting divorced; I was disillusioned with so much I had believed to be true; and old health problems were resurfacing. Only among the redwoods did I feel supported, held and nourished. The redwoods awakened the oldest part of my soul. They gave me the gift of "tree time," their own perception of time and longevity. If you have ever been in a redwood forest you have experienced this. There is a stillness, a silence among the trees that makes time slow down. It is a visceral reaction, where you feel your breath deepen, metabolism slow and muscles relax. If you haven't experienced tree time, it is time you did.

Responsibility and Reverence

We are all activists even if we don't see ourselves as such. Everyone has at least one thing that they are passionate about. There is something that brings us to rage or tears when we think of an injustice that is close to our hearts. For me, humanity's total lack of reverence for all other species on this planet upsets me the most. As much as I want humanity to thrive on this planet, my deepest concern is for the rest of the beings we share this miraculous Earth with. I know our survival depends on them much more than their survival on us. We have a responsibility to do our best, to reverse the damage we have created and continue to create on a daily basis. I speak to plants and I know they want us to continue our co-evolution with them, but we need to slow down, listen and remember.

Grandmother Tree

Although plants are autotrophic, and don't need humans to survive, we do provide some benefit, in both our spreading and hybridizing of their seeds and from our love and adoration. I have meditated with enough plants to know they love to be seen, appreciated and used for their healing qualities. Like us, they appreciate being noticed and praised for the gifts they provide.

There is a 2nd-growth redwood tree beside my house whom I call Grandmother Tree. I have been speaking to this tree since my husband and I bought the property where she lives. Grandmother Tree has one of the largest burls I've eve seen at her base. In this burl are the spirits of Green Man and an ancient tree fairy. I see them both very clearly, although it is with Green Man that I most often converse. Green Man has been called by many names: Shen Nong, Pan, and Osiris are but a few. He is one of the manifestations that nature speaks through. With Green Man and Grandmother Tree I have had the most profound insights about humanity's place in the natural world. I have listened to nature as she describes witnessing the demise of the human race. It is our mad quest for dominance that has separated us from the rest of Life and has stunted evolutionary growth as a result. Instead of working alongside nature, we have attempted to manipulate and control it, to the detriment of all of life on Earth.

The Earth is a living being with countless ecosystems that are always altered and sometimes destroyed by human habitation. The dramatic decrease in redwood trees has also decreased the intense fog that once engulfed and sustained life in the millions of acres of redwood canopy. The loss of canopy and fog has led to the decline of species within an ecosystem that has existed for millions of years. We can't foresee the consequences of destroying such an ecosystem.

Grandmother Tree has spoken to me about how humans have nearly destroyed themselves time and time again. She says we are a resilient species but not beyond extinction. Her neutrality soothes me. She is matter-of-fact. Her attitude says, *We enjoy having you here, but it's your choice to stay.* We can destroy or we can create, and we will reap what we sow. Life on Earth will thrive. The question is, will we?

One of my favorite conversations with Grandmother Tree came after a women's herbal symposium where I'd had an intimate conversation with a tiny little fir tree. After I told Grandmother Tree about my experiences, she spoke to me these words: *It is your responsibility to share our stories. You and others who listen have been chosen to speak for the plants. It is your responsibility to remind others that as interconnected species, we rely on each other, that we need each other to not only survive but to thrive. You must tell your human brothers and sisters the life we have to give. They have to remember that they depend on us to live.* I began to cry and I said, *I will tell as many people as I can and I will make sure that you will remain here forever.* She chuckled and said, *I won't be here forever and neither will you. And that's okay. That's not how it's meant to be.* Even after her words of insistence for the human race, I was still more concerned with her fate than our own.

I think about Grandmother Tree when I am away from my California home and I mourned her when I returned home last year and realized the top sixty feet of her canopy had blown down in a storm. As soon as I got out of the car I noticed the skyline was different but I couldn't place exactly what had changed. I walked out to the pond and looked toward the house. Instead of two towering redwoods among the trees I saw only one. The top of Grandmother Tree would have taken out our entire home if she had fallen in the opposite direction. I am grateful she did not. Tears came instantly when I entered the woods to find where the top had fallen. She had been an enormous tree and I said a prayer for all the life among her branches.

Redwood's Song

The beauty of redwoods is that they will regenerate indefinitely. The loss of even sixty feet will not kill Grandmother Tree. In the old-growth stumps that scatter the land, small redwood trees, huckleberries and ferns thrive. Life continues. Redwoods remind us that life goes on long after we are gone. They tell us that life is impermanent and precious and to remember what life is about: connection, reverence and love.

Think Back
Slow Down
Listen
Remember

Jessica Baker, LAc, RH (AHG)

Redwood Recipes

Redwood Needle Honey

Harvest enough tender new-growth redwood needles to fill a quart jar 3/4 full. Collect 1-2 cones if desired. Place needles and cones in the top of a double boiler and pour one quart of honey over needles. Infuse over low heat for 45 minutes, allowing water to evaporate off. Pour honey through muslin or cheesecloth and collect honey in a glass quart jar. Redwood honey is good to astringe and expectorate wet coughs and can be taken as a daily tonic to remind you to slow down and listen to your body's wisdom.

Conifer Rose Cordial

-   1/2 ounce redwood needles (or other conifer needles)
-   1/2 ounce rosehips
-   2 cups brandy
-   1 1/2 cups spring water
-   1 cup honey
-   rose water

Soak redwood needles and rosehips in brandy for 5 days. After 5 days, strain herbs and collect the alcohol in a glass bottle. Soak the strained herbs in spring water for 3 days. Strain herbs and collect the water. Warm the water and dissolve 1 cup honey into it. Combine the water/honey mixture with the alcohol extraction. Add a dash of rose water for a more floral taste. Stir well. Pour into a clean glass bottle and let sit for at least one month. As Diana De Luca, a medical herbalist from Sebastopol, California says, a cordial gets better with age, just like we do! Sip with friends as you gather to celebrate any occasion.

Redwood Respiratory Blend

Harvest tender needles of redwood and other conifers in your area. I love Douglas fir, pine (especially piñon and knotty pine), blue cedar, and cypress. Look around the bases of the trees and you may notice other medicinal herbs growing around them.

In the redwood forest I often find wild violet, self-heal (prunella), plantain and yarrow. Harvest the companion plants if they are safe for consumption. Collect enough needles and herbs to fill a quart jar 1/2 full.

Boil one quart of water and then pour over herbs. Let steep for 20-30 minutes (cover with lid to keep volatile oils from evaporating in the air). Strain off plant material and compost. Store tea in a glass quart jar. Drink 1/2 cup of warm tea as needed for wet coughs that accompany a cold or flu. Add redwood needle honey if desired.

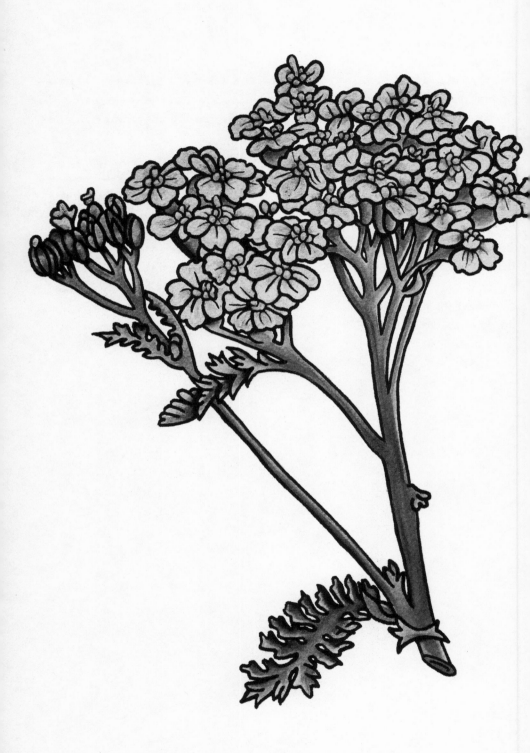

CHAPTER ELEVEN

Yarrow: Embrace Your Warrior Spirit

Yarrow
Achillea millefolium

- **Properties:** Spicy, Sweet, Cold
- **Meridians entered:** Lung, Liver, Spleen
- **Elements influenced:** Metal, Wood, Earth
- **Original habitat:** Native to temperate regions of the northern Hemisphere in Asia, Europe.
- **Habitats:** Coastal to alpine in disturbed soil, grasslands or open forest.

Description: Yarrow is a spreading perennial with green, aromatic, fern-like foliage and tiny white flowers in dense corymbs on stems rising 2-3 feet tall.

Embrace your warrior spirit
Gain your courageous heart

Traditional Herbalism

Yarrow is an herb for which I have a deep affinity. Since the first time I smelled and tasted yarrow in an herb class, I knew she was an ally of mine. Like the old saying goes: *Where the yarrow grows, there is one who knows.* It has been known as a witch's herb, a divination tool and a powerful medicine that is used in cultures spread far and wide. Yarrow has a circumboreal distribution, found throughout North America, Europe and Asia.

Although yarrow is known for many medicinal properties, like the ability to lower fever by diaphoresis and to stop bleeding, I use this curative plant when I need the courage to heal from any deep wound, be it physical or spiritual. With yarrow I am reminded of Achilles, the mythical warrior of Greek antiquity for whom *Achillea millefolium* is named. Achilles was not only handsome—and brutal—he was also known for his immense bravery and courage on and off the battlefield. His legendary ability to heal from injury is mirrored in his namesake plant.

Yarrow is a powerful vulnerary, and can stop internal and external bleeding. One of the concerns of an open wound is infection. Along with staunching the blood, yarrow is anti-bacterial and anti-microbial. While yarrow can close a wound, she can also protect from any bacteria that may have entered it.

According to seventeenth century herbalist and botanist Nicholas Culpeper, yarrow will "stop the terms [menstruation] in women, being boiled in wine and the decoction drank." Yarrow will also "stop the whites [leucorrhea] in women" and helps with gonorrhea in men. The healing nature of yarrow is so vast that it has been said to help with things from hair loss and toothache to healing severe wounds. The Shoshone boiled yarrow root for gas pains and a decoction of the tea was applied to boils and sores. In medieval Europe, people wore amulets of nettle and yarrow to allay fear and ward off negativity and seers drank yarrow tea prior to divination to enhance their powers of perception.

Upon inhalation, the aromatic properties of yarrow open the sinuses and allow for deeper breaths. The strong anti-bacterial and anti-microbial properties help with reducing respiratory infections. As a diaphoretic, yarrow is often blended with peppermint and elderflower as a safe herbal tea to reduce fevers in children. In Chinese medicine, the ability of aromatic plants, like yarrow, to open the mind make it a powerful medicine for bringing clarity to confused or disturbed thinking.

Yarrow sticks are the tools of divination for the *I-Ching* and the interpretation of their patterns reflects the disharmony the seeker has with his internal and external environment. The images created by the throwing of yarrow sticks are interpreted as one of the sixty-four hexagrams that influence much of Chinese philosophy. *Wu Xi* (shamans) and others who throw the *I-Ching* know how to interpret subtle patterns that may cause discomfort or disease within the body or spirit. A correct pattern diagnosis, along with the proper tools—herbs, manual therapies, mantras, and exercises—can aid in creating lasting change

Peaceful Warrior

To me, yarrow is a peaceful warrior. Its power is strong enough to stop the bleeding from a gunshot wound, yet safe enough to reduce a child's fever. This is the kind of medicine we need in these times when old wounds are resurfacing on a global scale. The suicide rate is at an all-time high and we are in a time of racial and religious conflict where violence is escalating at an alarming rate. We are fighting a personal war within and have chosen violence in response to the fear and guilt we feel for our part in the destruction around us. We all need the courage of yarrow to transform the global paradigm of violence.

For me personally, yarrow is an ally that helps me access my courageous warrior within, encouraging me to be an activist for those who can't speak for themselves. Yarrow has given me the courage to write this book, to speak for the trees, flowers and fungi that call to me. Yarrow provides the bravery for me to say that violence is not the answer. Yarrow tells me to use my voice and to offer alternate solutions to those who want to heal. Yarrow allows me to see the patterns within nature and within myself to find the answers I am looking for.

Once our patterns of behavior are placed before us, we have a choice of whether or not to change the circumstances that cause us to react. Interpreting the *I-Ching* or listening to the voice within us will guide us toward what needs to be resolved to move forward. Changing course or altering our belief systems can be very scary. Yarrow is here to remind us that we have the strength to overcome anything, that we can alter the course of our lives and find balance in that decision.

Yarrow's Song

My meditations with yarrow have been profound. On backpacking trips I have gathered wild yarrow many times and made sun infusions to drink along the walk. I feel instantly cooled and invigorated and I have a clarity that makes all life around me come into greater focus. I feel awakened to colors, sounds and sensations. With each sip I feel sharper and more aware. I have more stamina and I feel deeply connected to all around me.

Yarrow grows all over my property in California and I have found the combination of wild yarrow and wild rose to provide that balance of courage and self-love all warriors need when confronted with hard decisions. Yarrow accesses your courage, while rose helps you lead from your heart. This combination encourages the compassion and patience needed to make wise decisions. I use the two together when both a clear head and an open heart are needed.

Embrace your warrior spirit
Gain your courageous heart

Yarrow Recipes

Cool Yourself Tea

Mix 1/4 ounce each of the following dried herbs: yarrow flowers, elder flowers, peppermint leaves and lemon balm leaves. Store in a glass jar. Steep 1 tbsp. of herbs in 8 ounces of boiled water. Strain out herbs and drink as needed to reduce fever in children or adults. Bundle up while drinking the hot tea. Add honey if desired.

Divine Meditation

Diffuse 2 drops yarrow essential oil, 2 drops frankincense, and 2 drops myrrh in a water-based aromatherapy diffuser. As the aroma envelops the room, close your eyes, inhale deeply and allow yourself to relax. When your breath deepens, focus on a situation where you have a hard time finding a peaceful solution. What emotions come up as you think of this person/scenario? As these emotions come to the surface, breathe deeply and let them pass. After confronting these emotions, what sensations do you feel in your body?

Whatever you are feeling—anger, grief, fear—release it through breath, tears, or chanting. Let it go in any way that feels right for you. With each inhalation, fill yourself up with a golden divine light. Allow this light, this shower of *Qi*, to engulf every cell of your body and filter out into the energy fields around you. Breathe deeply into your lower abdomen until you feel grounded and are ready to open your eyes and integrate back into your day.

Courageous Warrior Spritzer

- 1 ounce spring water
- 4 drops yarrow essential oil
- 3 drops fir (or any conifer) essential oil
- 2 drops rose (or rose geranium) essential oil

Blend essential oils and spring water in a glass spritzer bottle. Shake well and mist yourself when you need strength, courage and compassion for yourself and others in a difficult situation. Breathe in compassion and love and breathe out hatred and violence. Take three intentional breaths and communicate from a place of benevolence. This essential oil blend is also great to diffuse in a conference or meeting room where important decisions are made.

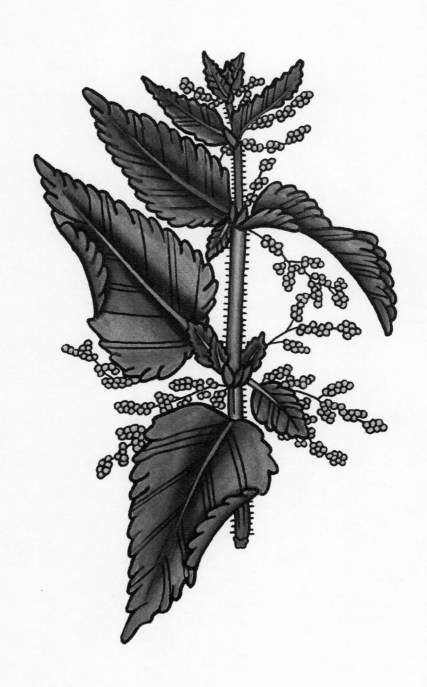

CHAPTER TWELVE

Nettle: Pay Attention

Urtica dioica
Stinging Nettle
Qian Ma

- **Properties:** Salty, Bland, Slightly Spicy, Cool
- **Meridians entered:** Liver, Lung, Urinary Bladder
- **Elements influenced:** Wood, Metal, Water
- **Original habitat:** Cooler regions of northern Europe, Asia and North America.
- **Habitats:** Found in temperate climates with plentiful sunlight; areas of high nitrogen.

Description: Nettles are dioecious herbaceous perennials that can grow up to 4-5 feet tall. The soft heart-spaced leaves are opposite, serrated, dark green and covered in stinging and non-stinging hairs. The tiny white flowers are in elongated clusters towards the top of the stem.

Pay attention
Heed the call

Evolution Through Irritation

Life is prickly. It can burn and sting; it can irritate us to the point of thinking we are going to lose it. Just like nettle. And like nettle, life nurtures us deep down to the cellular level. "Pay attention," nettles say when you brush past them in a hurry. "Pay attention, you know what you need to do."

Nettle was one of the first plants I met when I started studying herbalism. A favorite in the Northern California herb scene, it grows abundantly and is so full of vital nutrients that it became a staple for me as a vegetarian. The nutrient profile for nettle is impressive. A hundred grams of blanched nettles provides 40% of the recommended allowance of vitamin A, 48% calcium, 39% manganese, 14% magnesium, 9% iron and 5% protein. A hundred grams seems like a lot until you think about making nettle pesto or nettle lasagna.

The vigor you experience from an infusion of freshly harvested nettle is like that of Popeye with his spinach. Except you don't want to fight—instead you feel like you could go climb a mountain. Until you have harvested your own food from the wild it is hard to imagine how you feel afterward. Forget being bloated, tired and sluggish. Imagine instead feeling vital, nourished like you've never been before. This is how you feel after eating or drinking nettles. Nettle reminds us to pay attention to what is most important to our physical bodies: our health. What we consume directly affects our physical, mental and spiritual well-being. Nettles not only nourish us with micronutrients, calcium and amino acids, they also nourish us by encouraging us to make the best choices for our personal evolutions.

Himalayan Medicine

In 2000 I went to Nepal during the Mayashivaratra, the annual Hindu festival in honor of Shiva, to visit a college friend, Arun. My trip wasn't a popular choice at the time, as my boyfriend (now husband) couldn't go and wanted me to wait for him. I didn't want to wait for him. I felt this was my chance and if I didn't go then I might not make it for years. I'm grateful I went when I did. At that time, Gorkha, where I traveled to meet Arun, and the other towns in the region were already under a six o'clock curfew because of Maoist activity and I could feel the tension rising between the Maoists, the government and the citizens. Coming events would change the lives of all Nepalis, including Arun's family.

The first couple of days in Kathmandu I spent visiting temples and trying to score as much hash as I could. If you've ever traveled to Nepal or India, especially if you've gone alone, you know that you will have more people than you ever wanted trying to help you out. They want to show you this shop, take you to this restaurant, have you meet their relatives—the list goes on and on. For me it was draining, irritating and also exhilarating. With the help of strangers I was reunited with my old friend, attended a wedding, and taken to places I didn't even know existed. One of these strangers, a guide named Krishna, took me hiking outside of Pokhara in the Annapurna Mountains. Besides seeing the *sadhus* at the temples, I was most excited about going backpacking in the mountains. My experience was not quite what I expected. But life never really is.

Krishna and I had only been hiking for a couple of hours when I started feeling hot, nauseous and dizzy. I was getting slow and clumsy and couldn't even enjoy the beauty around me. My frustration began to grow as I realized that I was going to have to ask Krishna to stop. He was used to hiking this trail, as he had done so often with other tourists, so he thought maybe the elevation was starting to affect me. I was afraid the water I'd drunk at the Newari wedding I attended was beginning to revisit me. I knew it hadn't been advisable to drink the offered jug water, but I thought what the hell, since I had already been served food on a plate blessed in water. I was also hoping the homemade *raksi* would kill off any bacteria or protozoa I might have been drinking. It did not.

Once my ego let up and I told Krishna I had to stop, I took off my too-heavy backpack and began to look around. I took in all the beauty of the majestic scenery and decided to take some pictures. Among intense stomach cramps, I clicked away at my Olympus camera. Oblivious to what was behind me, I stepped back and felt my entire sweat-soaked back burn with an intensity I haven't felt before. I whipped my head around and saw the biggest nettle plant I've ever seen. I'm used to seeing nettles in bunches, like a hedge. This was one plant, at least two feet wide and five feet tall. As my back stung and burned and I glared at the vicious nettle, I heard the nettle plant say clearly, *Pay attention. You know what you need to do.* I was still in shock from the stinging and the cramping was becoming unbearable, so I didn't quite understand at the time. Once the burning subsided, Krishna and I walked the rest of the way to the first village to spend the night. As I lay on my cot and had a chance to replay the day and my frustration with myself for being so slow on the trail, I thought, "Yes, I do know what I need to do." The next morning I told Krishna I had to turn around and go back to Kathmandu, where I spent the next few days on the toilet.

During my visit to Nepal I spent a glorious four days in the country home of Arun's parents. The home was in Chitwan, and was more than an acre of rice, mangos, pineapples, and vegetables overlooking the river. I spent most of the time being nursed back to health by Arun's mom. Feeding me nothing but jasmine tea and ghee soup with bland vegetables and rice, my gut and spirit recovered as I sat in the pavilion and watched the river roll by.

I'm glad I went to Nepal when I did. Otherwise I would not have been able to visit their country home. In June 2001, the massacre of the Nepali royal family occurred in the Narayanhity Royal Palace in the capital city, Kathmandu. Once this occurred, a country already ridden with corrupt politicians and civil unrest just got worse. A year-long media blackout didn't help the situation and further secluded Nepal from the outside world. During this period, Arun's parents home in Chitwan was fire-bombed. They were forced to evacuate and to this day haven't been able to go back to their ancestral home.

Pay attention, you know what you need to do. I am grateful that Arun and his family paid attention; they listened to their instincts and left their home before anyone got injured or killed in the bombing.

Traditional Medicine

Nettle is one of our circumboreal plants, which means it inhabits the forested temperate regions of North American and Eurasia. For millennia, nettle has been used for food and medicine, and along with hemp and flax, has been used around the world to make textiles. Evidence from 2,800 years ago shows that nettle fiber was being imported into Denmark for textile products, even though the area had robust flax production at the time. Giant nettle was one of the plants used in the Himalayas for weaving cloth, and can be found in tombs dating from 400 BC-50 CE.

Nettle's use a medical herb is also found throughout time. In Algeria, nettles are powdered and mixed with powdered jasmine for gonorrhea. Seventeenth-century herbalist Nicolas Culpeper has a lot to say about nettles. He writes, "Mars claims dominion over nettles," and that "eating metal tops in the spring expels the phlegmatic superfluities from the body, which the coldness and moisture of winter have left behind." This is why eating spring nettle greens are so important to Western herbalists. Nettle helps shake off the sluggishness of winter. In *Culpeper's Herbal* the decoction of the leaves in wine is said to be very effective against "diseases of the female sex." A water decoction of the seeds promotes urination and expels gravel and stones from the kidneys and urinary tract. Many other uses are described such as treatments for gangrene, fistulas, scabs and itching.

The nettle seed decoction has been used in a curious manner since at least the time of ancient Greeks. It was used as a remedy against the sting of venomous creatures, the bite of a mad dog, and the poisonous quality of mushrooms, hemlock, henbane, nightshade, mandrake, and other herbs that alter the senses. Culpeper writes that for bites and stings, one should rub nettle seed decoction and a little salt into the forehead and temples and into the injuries, and also drink the decoction.

In Chinese herbalism, nettle is known as *Qian Ma*. The flavor is salty, bland, and slightly sweet. The nature is cool and has an affinity to go to the Liver, Lung and the Urinary Bladder. Nettle treats damp accumulation anywhere in the body. It is used particularly for the water retention that creates urinary difficulties, edema, and joint stiffness. When dampness accumulates, obstruction of the meridians can occur, causing pain and lack of mobility of the joints. This is why nettle is known in various cultures as a remedy for pain and stiffness of the joints.

Nettle is cool, astringent and nourishing to the blood and can be helpful for treating mid-cycle spotting, excessive menstrual bleeding and even bleeding in the stool. It is of utmost importance, of course, to get a diagnosis of the cause of any excessive bleeding. Nettle is effective for stopping bleeding due to a blood deficiency or when there is heat entering the blood.

In my clinical practice, I work with nettles from a Western herbalist perspective. Western herbalists regard nettles as a highly nutritious spring tonic rich in vital minerals. They, along with dandelion and yellow dock, are the best combination to celebrate the start of spring. The bitter flavor stimulates digestion and clears out the dampness that can manifest after a winter of eating heavier, harder-to-digest foods. The high mineral content contributes to nettle's medicinal effect, but also has a diuretic effect.

I would caution against the excessive use of nettles in those who take diuretic drugs. Overall, I have found nettles to be one of the most important plants in my *materia medica*. Nettle grows abundantly, is delicious when cooked, and is one of the most densely nutritive medicinal plants I know of.

Nettle's Song

Nettle is an intriguing plant. Nourishing and clearing, stimulating and astringing, nettle seems to know exactly what your body needs and then provides it. Once the nutrients and minerals in nettle begin to nourish your mind, tissues, and organs, awareness begins to spark. You begin to discern what is serving you and what is not. You make choices based on what will nurture and support you.

> *Pay attention*
> *Heed the call*

Nettle Recipes

Nourishing Nettle Tea

- 1 ounce dried nettles
- 1 ounce dried milky oats
- 1 ounce dried raspberry leaf
- 1 ounce dried linden blossoms

Mix all herbs together. Take 1-2 tsp. and add to 8 ounces boiled water. Steep for 15-20 minutes. Strain off herbs and drink infusion slowly.

Concentrated Chlorophyll

Juice fresh nettle tops in a wheatgrass juicer. Take 1 ounce nettle juice daily. Drink 8 ounces of water afterward.

Poison Oak Poultice

- 1/2 ounce dried nettles
- 1/2 ounce dried manzanita leaves
- 1/2 ounce dried Oregon grape root

Powder all ingredients in an herb grinder. Moisten with water, apple cider vinegar and/or witch hazel. Apply to poison oak. Let sit on skin for at least 20 minutes and rinse gently with cool water.

PART IV

Adulthood/Wisdom Plants

Angelica, Hawthorn, Rosemary, Reishi

Now that I'm in my early forties and have cultivated my connection with plants for almost half my life, I am a different person. I am happy, healthy, and have long, deep relationships with human and plant kin. The love and connection I feel is because of the gifts of the plants, because I listened when the plants spoke to me. I am still growing, sometimes slowly and steadily, sometime in leaps and bounds that always leave me exhilarated, alive, and a little wiser. My journey with plants, with Mother Earth, and with myself will continue to evolve and deepen as I sit and listen to the songs of the plants.

In Part IV, I chose angelica, for showing me my divinity; hawthorn, for opening my heart; rosemary, for reminding me; and reishi, for going deep.

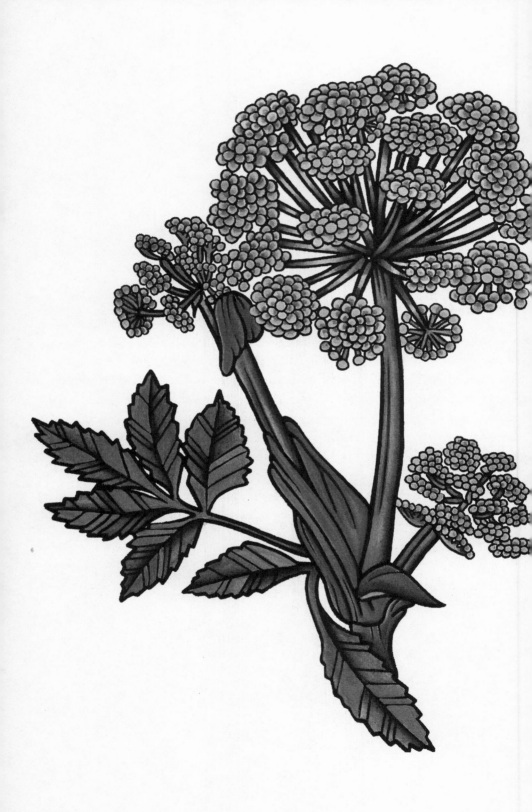

CHAPTER THIRTEEN

Angelica: Hear Your Divinity

Angelica sinensis
Dang Gui (Dong Quai)

- **Properties:** Sweet, Spicy, Warm
- **Meridians entered:** Heart, Liver, Spleen
- **Elements influenced:** Fire, Wood, Earth
- **Original habitat:** East Asia to China.
- **Habitats:** Highly cultivated for its medicinal properties; hardy to most zones.

Angelica dahurica
Bai Zhi

- **Properties:** Spicy, Warm
- **Meridians entered:** Lung, Stomach, Spleen
- **Elements influenced:** Metal, Earth
- **Original habitat:** Siberia, eastern Russia, Mongolia, NE China, Japan, Korea, Taiwan
- **Habitats:** Highly cultivated in Sichuan province of China.

Angelica pubescens
Du Huo

- **Properties:** Spicy, Bitter, Warm
- **Meridians entered:** Liver, Kidney, Urinary Bladder
- **Elements influenced:** Wood, Water
- **Original habitat:** Temperate to subarctic regions of Northern Hemisphere.
- **Habitats:** Highly cultivated in China; hardy to most zones.

Angelica archangelica
Angelica, or Garden Angelica

- **Properties:** Spicy, Bitter, Warm
- **Meridians entered:** Lung, Kidney, Urinary Bladder
- **Elements influenced:** Metal, Water
- **Original habitat:** North, NE Europe, Russia, Iceland, Greenland, Himalayas.
- **Habitats:** Northern temperate regions

Description: Angelicas are biennial plants that produce compound leaves the first year and a strong hollow stem up to 6 feet tall or more. Large clusters of white umbel flower appear the second year. The large yellow-green leaves are compound, biternate with inflated stem bases. The lower leaves can be 2-3 feet long with toothed leaflets. All plants in the *Apiacea* family look very similar. Proper identification is necessary before harvesting any plants in this family.

Listen closely
Hear your divinity

Chinese Herbalism

The genus *Angelica* is varied in its medicinal uses. Angelica can help with a variety of conditions like back pain, headache from sinus congestion, and anemia. Angelica is named after the angels and has been used in purification against evil influences. From prevention of contagious diseases to menstrual regulation, angelica is an essential and powerful medicine.

In Chinese herbalism we use several different species of angelica as medicine. It is very important to know which variety you are using because they can have very different actions within the body. The most common preparation is called *Dang Gui Pian* and is used to treat painful or lack of menstruation, pain and spasms, and constipation. The root of *Angelica sinensis*, *Dang Gui*, means "state of return" and is known as a popular women's herb. In truth, *Dang Gui* goes way deeper than helping with painful menstrual cramps. She is a master herb that can both nourish and invigorate the blood. This quality of nourishing the blood allows for its use in reducing pain in blood-deficient people who may be weakened or easily fatigued by blood-invigorating herbs. When there is blood deficiency, pain and spasms may arise from a lack of nourishment to the muscles and tissues. The action of nourishing the blood implies a warming quality, so *Dang Gui* can help with abdominal pain related to blood deficiency and coldness.

Dang Gui can also treat traumatic injuries, especially in conjunction with blood-activating herbs, which speed up the healing of bruises, fractured or broken bones, and swelling and injuries of the tendons. Its nourishing nature can also treat the constipation due to dryness that is common in the elderly, women in postpartum, or in anyone in the late or recovery stages of chronic disease.

Other conditions that may affect health and well-being can be treated with *Dang Gui*. The root is divided into the head of the rhizome, called *Dang Gui Tou*, which treats headaches due to blood deficiency, and the small roots that come off of the main root, called *Dang Gui Wei*, which are used to treat pain and numbness in the extremities due to blood deficiency. Used together, *Dang Gui Pian*, *Dang Gui Tou*, and *Dang Gui Wei* can treat pain and spasms of the entire body and can be a powerful medicine for debilitated people.

Angelica dahurica, or *Bai Zhi*, is used to treat headaches due to external wind and cold invading the meridians. This angelica also dispels cold from the meridians and body and relieves pain along the stomach channel. This association with the stomach channel makes it useful in treating frontal headaches, pain around the eyes, toothaches and nasal obstructions. You can also treat diarrhea and leucorrhea because *Bai Zhi* will dispel dampness from the lower *Jiao*, which includes the large intestine, urinary bladder, kidneys and reproductive organs.

Angelica pubescens is known as *Du Huo*, which translates to "self-reliant existence." Like *Angelica dahurica, Du Huo* dispels wind and dampness to relieve pain. *Du Huo* specifically treats pain and weakness of the lower back and knees. Sometimes lower back and knee pain are attributed to kidney yang deficiency. These pains may increase when there is cold and dampness and there can be sensitivity to cold temperatures, drinks or food. *Du Ho* can also treat headaches and the sensations of heaviness in the head and muscles that accompany a cold or flu.

Traditional and Modern Knowledge

In laboratory studies *Angelica sinensis* has been shown to be effective both at stimulating and inhibiting the smooth muscle of the uterus. When the uterus is in a state of relaxation, *A. sinensis* can induce contraction, and if the uterus is in a contracted state, then it promotes relaxation. This dual action allows the herb to both relieve spasms and stop pain.

In Western herbalism, *Angelica archangelica* is governed by the Sun in Leo and should only be gathered at this time. *A. archangelica* is said to resist poison by defending and comforting the heart, blood and spirits. The powder of the root, when added to distilled water, cleanses out wounds and helps them heal faster. Distilled water of angelica improves eyesight. Angelica root taken in the morning before breakfast helps the body protect itself from the evil of pestilent air. Culpeper also talks about linen soaked in angelica-infused vinegar. He says to put a bit of the soaked cloth inside a lemon or an orange skin, and to prick holes in the skin and smell the medicinal vinegar as a way to protect yourself from epidemic diseases. Traditional and modern herbalists agree that *Angelica archangelica* protects against poison, pestilent factors and epidemics. She is an effective painkiller and is used for women in labor, toothache, and pain from gout and sciatica.

Angelic Medicine

Angelica archangelica has spiritual properties as well. The root of *Angelica archangelica* helps you see your guardian angels and hear the wisdom they have to impart. In *Culpeper's Herbal*, the author admits he doesn't know why angelica was named, but he postulates that the name was given to man by the ministry of an angel. The medicinal qualities of angelica are here to safeguard our bodies and souls, which is the same reason God made angels.

Some aromatherapists use angelica essential oil on clients near the moment of death to help them to hear the angels calling them home. The passing is said to be peaceful, with a feeling of joyfulness at hearing and feeling the presence of angels.

Angelica Meditations

My personal experience with using angelica in meditation and purification has been deeply healing. On one occasion, I was sitting by my tent at the Women's Herbal Symposium and I crushed some dried angelica root that I had harvested years earlier into small pieces. I chewed on a small piece and lit some of the powdered root on fire. As I inhaled her aroma my spiritual guides instantly surrounded me. I was completely held in their embrace and I felt as if I was hovering over my own body and looking down upon myself as these loving beings did. I saw myself, my struggles, my strengths; I saw my true self and I felt a love for myself that can only come from benevolence. Once the incense burned out I was back in my body, sitting on the Earth, feeling completely at peace.

Angelica's Song

I think about the name angelica and wonder whether God(dess) made the virtues of this plant known to man by the ministry of an angel, as Culpeper states. I like to imagine that angels are ministering spirits, here to safeguard of our souls and our bodies. Angelica helps move the divine through us, allowing us to see the light within ourselves.

Listen closely
Hear your divinity

Angelica Recipes

Dang Gui Jin

Decoct 1 ounce of dried *Dang Gui* in 1 quart of water for 30 minutes. Strain out *Dang Gui* and add 2-3 cups honey to warm *Dang Gui* tea. Mix liquids well. Take 1 tbsp. 2-3 times daily to nourish blood, stop pain or regulate menstruation.

Angelica Incense

Powder 1 *Angelica archangelica* root. Burn a pinch of the root on charcoal to invoke your guardian angels. Thank them for their presence, wisdom and compassion.

Spirit of the Sages Spritzer

- 3 drops white sage essential oil
- 3 drops clary sage essential oils
- 3 drops *Angelica archangelica* essential oil

Add essential oils to 1 ounce spring water. Mix well and put in a glass spritzer bottle. Mist yourself as needed for clarity, relaxation, and meditation.

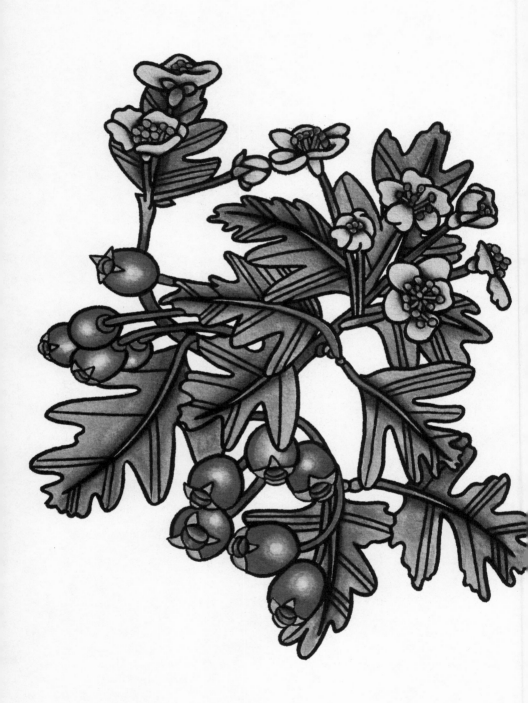

CHAPTER FOURTEEN

Hawthorn: Open Your Heart

Crataegus laevigata
Hawthorn berry
Shan Zha

- **Properties:** Sweet, Sour, Slightly Warm
- **Meridians entered**: Liver, Spleen, Stomach, Heart
- **Elements influenced**: Wood, Earth
- **Original habitat**: Temperate regions of Northern Hemisphere in Europe, Asia, N. America.
- **Habitats**: Temperate regions across the world.

Crataegus oxyacantha
Hawthorn, Haw

- **Properties:** Sweet, Sour, Slightly Warm
- **Meridians entered**: Heart, Spleen, Liver
- **Elements influenced**: Fire, Earth
- **Original habitat**: Temperate regions of Northern Hemisphere in Europe, Asia, N. America.
- **Habitats**: Temperate regions across the world.

Description: Hawthorn are deciduous trees that can grow to be up to 50 feet tall. Green leaves with lobed or serrated edges that vary in size grow off of mostly thorny stems. Fragrant 5-petaled white flowers grow in clusters. In fall there are bright red edible berries.

Open your heart
Let the transformation begin

Open Gently

Everyone wants to be cracked open. We experiment with drugs and psychedelic substances to blow our minds wider than we even though imaginable. We play football, skydive and speed in our cars for the excitement and the rush. We watch death and destruction as entertainment and participate in violent computer simulations until the domestic violence and world wars of our reality no longer bothers us. We obsessively check our social media status to see if we're liked, followed and adored. For those addicted or crippled from these activities, they know what they're doing to themselves, yet they can't stop. We all hear the voice inside our heads that says, "Stop hurting yourself; you're better than this; get off the computer and go outside." We are addicted to countless substances, excessive behavior, and social media. It is wreaking havoc on our nervous systems.

When I envision a person cracked open it is a red-faced cartoon character with his head blown open like a volcano erupting. He is not necessarily angry, but there is so much pressure—social, financial, marital—that just like a volcano, the only way to release the build-up is to explode. Explosions can come in the form of binge gaming, drinking, eating or intense emotional outbursts. When I begin to feel this way, I reach for hawthorn. Hawthorn has a way of cracking you open gently, lovingly, and in the timing that is right for you.

Chinese Herbalism

The best herb I work with to support digestion and transform emotional release is *Shan Zha*, hawthorn berries. The nature of *Shan Zha* is sweet, sour and slightly warming. The berries enter into the spleen and the stomach and eliminate stagnation from the digestion, helping to reduce abdominal fullness, distention, pain, and diarrhea. They are especially effective if one eats heavy meats or oily, fatty foods.

Although I usually combine them in a formula, I have had great results with a simple tincture of hawthorn berries for those who have a tendency to eat to the point of feeling stuffed. A popular folk formula for grief, heartache, or melancholy is a combination of mimosa bark (*He Huan Pi* – eternal happiness bark), rose, and hawthorn leaves and flowers. For those who also experience digestive upset with an emotional response, I like to add hawthorn berries to

125

transform and eliminate dampness, and milky oats to strengthen digestion and relax the nervous system.

More and more research shows ingestion of hawthorn berries reduces plaque in the arteries and has a tonic effect on the cardiac muscles. Hawthorn berries also activate blood circulation, so they can help with blood stagnation, which can manifest as postpartum abdominal pain, amenorrhea (lack of menstruation), and cardiac disorders. The blood-moving properties of hawthorn berries make them a great herb to treat cardiovascular disorders like hypertension, angina, and high cholesterol. Research posted in the *Journal of Traditional Chinese Medicine* has shown that a two-week course of treatment with powdered extract of *Shan Zha* (hawthorn berry) and *Mai Ya* (barley sprout) reduced hyperlipidemia in 92% of the participants (127 patients). In another study of hawthorn berries, this time in conjunction with other herbs, triglyceride levels and serum cholesterol dropped by 87% in almost 81% of participants. Hawthorn berries have also demonstrated and inhibitory effect against staphylococcus, salmonella, E. coli, and pseudomonas.

Hawthorn does enhance the activity of the cardiac drug digoxin, it should be noted. Anyone on digoxin or ingesting plants that contain cardiac glycosides, such as *Digitalis* species or *Convallaria majalis*, should avoid the use of hawthorn or make sure their use is closely monitored by a competent practitioner. The coronary vasodilating and antiarrhythmic effects of hawthorn can affect the dosage needed for certain heart conditions.

Transformational Medicine

The transformative properties of hawthorn berry are described and illustrated in multiple research studies, but to me that's not always as important as how ingesting the plant makes you feel. The more I work with hawthorn, the more I notice that the herb's ability to aid with the digestion of fats and heavy foods also applies to the digestion of unpleasant truths or emotions. Hawthorn berries work on the digestion, and specifically the spleen's function of transforming and transporting nutrients, which allows for *Yi* (idea) to bring clarity to the *Shen* (spirit).

In Chinese medicine, there is an intrinsic connection between digestion, emotions, and heart health. The spleen, a component of the digestive system, stores the *Yi*, which is represented by an ideogram that consists of two characters:

one for heart, and the other the musical note or sound "yin." Together, the characters describe the heart's ability to express itself through sounds, thoughts, or actions. *Yi* is responsible for all thoughts and ideas on an intellectual level. The ability to study, concentrate, and memorize is governed by how well *Yi* functions. Our *Shen* (spirit) is housed in the heart and is responsible for intimacy, cognition, intelligence, and consciousness. *Shen* governs our mental and emotional activities, our capacity to judge, and sleep. When our *Shen* is disturbed by thoughts of bills, war, or illness, our organs begin to work harder to keep homeostasis within the body.

Hawthorn slows down this state, allowing us to get into a state of relaxation, a place where we no longer need to focus on survival. Once there is cohesion between the *Shen* and the *Yi*, we have the space to reflect on our own consciousness and our places in the world. Hawthorn brings mental and emotional clarity, permitting the discovery of truths as your heart and mind unwind. This connection between hawthorn and the heart are found around the world.

Heart Medicine

While hawthorn berries have immense healing properties, the leaves and flowers of hawthorn have also long been used as a cardiac tonic. Strong enough to regulate heartbeat and reduce cardiac pain, but gentle enough to be used long-term without damaging any system in the body, hawthorn leaves and flowers are mentioned throughout history. In *Culpeper's Herbal*, Culpeper writes that the berries or the seeds in the berries beaten to a powder and drunk with wine are a singular remedy for dropsy (edema). Culpeper also mentions that the flowers and the seeds, bruised and boiled, will give instant relief of tormenting pain of the body. Tormenting pain makes me think that the sufferer is not only in physical pain, but in emotional and spiritual pain as well. Matthew Wood, in his book *The Earthwise Herbal*, discusses the use of hawthorn in children and adults with attention deficit disorder (ADD). For ADD, he uses hawthorn to increase focus and decrease irritability and nervousness.

In Britain, pollen counts show the presence of hawthorn before 6,000 BC. Celts honor hawthorn as the tree of Brigid, goddess of healing, childbirth, poetry, and smith craft. These attributes are connected to the heart and the fire element, as it takes a pure heart to heal, fiery passion to write poetry, and literal fire to forge metal. Brigid's connection to fire is so strong that a perpetual fire, believed to have burned until the sixteen century, was relit in 1993 at Kildare in her honor. Furthering the connection to fire, Culpeper attributes hawthorn to being under the rule of Mars (the fire planet). In Chinese medicine, the Fire element is associated with the heart, spirit, consciousness, speech, and sexuality. Our vitality and passion for life is reflected in the brilliance of our internal fire.

Hawthorn Healing

My personal experiences with hawthorn have been beautiful. As a budding herbalist I was only exposed to the medicinal properties of hawthorn leaf and flower. What really stuck with me was hawthorn for heartache and grief. For years I religiously made tea with hawthorn leaves and flowers, rose buds, milky oats, violets, and self-heal. I knew I needed to heal from some serious grief, as the feeling of intense loss still permeated my core. From my daily intake of this herbal brew, I began to transform all the dense energy of grief, anger, and fear that had been such a large part of my life. My anxiety greatly reduced and I felt lighter, brighter, and free. A spark ignited within me and I could see the world for the beautiful miracle it is.

Once I started adding the berries to the leaf and flower, I noticed a deeper shift. Not only did I notice a significant difference in my emotions and visceral reaction to stress, I also felt the inherent need to truly nurture myself. The transformative properties of hawthorn berries brought clarity to the ways I was still engaged in self-defeating thoughts and actions. *Shan Zha* cleared out the burdens and bridged the connection between the *Shen* and the *Yi*. Hawthorn medicine is still one of my (almost) daily allies for digestion, cardiac health, and my psyche.

Hawthorn's Song

Hawthorn's association with the heart and fire element in different cultures reminds us that our connection with hawthorn goes far deeper than we remember. The stories and lore of plants have shaped our psyche, culture, beliefs, and virtually every aspect of our existence. Hawthorn guides us back to our hearts, enlightens us to who we are, and helps us transform into our most magnificent selves. The combination of the leaves, flowers, and berries reminds us to love ourselves through all stages of life.

Open your heart
Let the transformation begin

Hawthorn Recipes

Happy Hawthorn Tea

- 1 ounce dried hawthorn flowers and leaves
- 1 ounce dried hawthorn berries
- 1 ounce dried rose buds
- 1 ounce dried lemon balm

Mix herbs together and store in a cool, dry place. Take 1 tbsp. herbs and steep in hot water for 15 minutes. Strain out herbs and drink 1 cup of tea slowly to lighten the heart and uplift the spirits.

Shan Zha Cordial

Fill a glass pint jar 1/2 full of hawthorn berries and citrus peel. Add one vanilla bean. Fill the rest of the jar with brandy. Let herbs infuse in brandy for 4 weeks. Strain off herbs and store infused brandy in a glass jar. Take 1 ounce of cordial as needed to help digest a heavy meal or drink with friends in celebration.

Brigid's Blend

- 1 ounce dried hawthorn flowers and leaves
- 1 ounce dried red raspberry leaf
- 2 ounces dried vitex berries
- 2 ounces dried rose petals

Mix herbs together and store in a cool, dry place. Take 1 tbsp. herbs and steep in hot water for 15 minutes. Strain out herbs and drink 1 cup of tea slowly to help regulate menstruation, tonify the uterus, and nourish the body after childbirth.

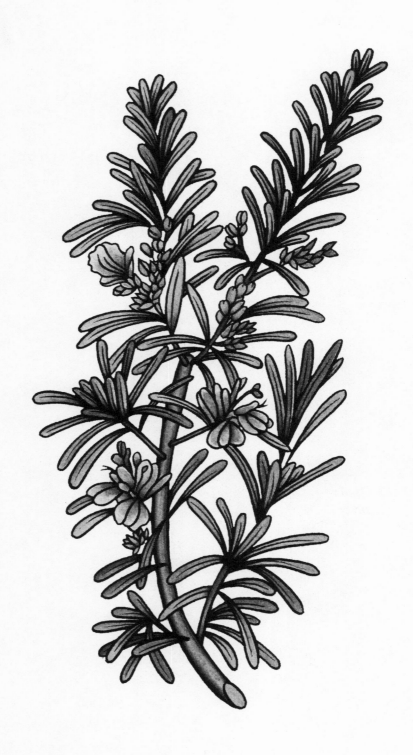

CHAPTER FIFTEEN

Rosemary: Remember Who You Are

Rosmarinus officinalis
Rosemary

- **Properties:** Spicy, Warm
- **Meridians entered:** Heart, Lungs, Spleen, Kidney
- **Elements influenced:** Fire, Metal, Earth, Water
- **Original habitat:** Mediterranean and Asia
- **Habitats:** Loves being by the sea in a moderate climate. She is reasonably hardy to cool temperatures and is drought tolerant.

Description: Rosemary is an evergreen shrub that can grow to be 6 feet tall. The aromatic needle-like leaves are gray-green on woody branches. The flowers are tiny and two-lipped, pale blue or purple to white.

Remember who you are
Be who you are meant to be

Traditional Herbalism

For me rosemary is like an internal cleansing bath. Rosemary clears out the gunk that holds me back from seeing my true potential. I credit rosemary with helping me move through some of the most painful experiences of my life. Going deep within myself and connecting to my radiance has been the scariest—and most rewarding—practice I have cultivated. There is so much in society that tells us we are unworthy, dirty sinners, so we need an ally like rosemary to remind us of how righteous and pure we are.

Rosmarinus, or "dew of the sea," named for the essential oils that rise to the tip of its needles when warmed by the coastal sun, has been revered for its medicine and aroma for thousands of years. As an herb that was medicinal, beautiful, and could grow in various environments, rosemary was widely traded and cultivated by the Greeks. The connection between remembrance and rosemary predates Greek antiquity, but it is from Greek physician and botanist Pedanius Dioscorides that we learn of rosemary as a symbol of commemoration and love. The essence of those qualities has endured through the centuries, elevating rosemary to the status of wisdom herb as she continues to capture hearts and minds.

Although rosemary has been used medicinally and cosmetically since antiquity, the herb is used in the United States of America mostly as a culinary spice. We are missing out on all of the wisdom and medicine rosemary has to offer. Like most spices, rosemary is carminative and can help reduce dyspepsia, fatigue, bloating, and flatulence after eating. Distilled water of rosemary, along with cloves, mace, cinnamon and anise seeds, can be drunk to freshen the breath. Rosemary is added to meats and vegetables not only for flavor, but as an aid to reduce the indigestion, bloating and fatigue that can accompany eating fats and uncooked vegetables. Rosemary is also known to many as an herb that will stimulate follicle growth for hair loss. It is present in cosmetic and hair products throughout the world, and consumers have been assured that using rosemary products will prevent premature balding. Even if this is true, rosemary is much more important than that.

In Western herbalism, we talk about rosemary as a circulatory tonic, not only to aid digestion and memory, but also to help with varicose veins and other signs of poor circulation. Rosemary's invigorating nature arouses the senses and stimulates *Qi* and blood flow to all the organs and extremities. As *Qi* and blood move freely throughout our bodies, our organs and minds are being pumped with new life force. We are not only physically stronger, because rosemary stimulates metabolism and aids in the assimilation of blood sugars and fat, but also more relaxed, because of its calming effect on the sympathetic nervous system. Nicolas Culpeper wrote about the added benefit of exercising after taking a decoction of rosemary to further enhance the circulatory properties.

Chinese Herbalism

Culpeper quotes Dioscorides as saying "that if a decoction [of rosemary] be made thereof with water, and they that have the yellow jaundice, exercise their bodies directly after the taking thereof, it will certainly cure them." We know that jaundice has to do with the function of the liver. In Chinese medicine, the sour flavor is associated with the Wood element, which corresponds to the liver and gallbladder, both of which play a huge role in our emotions, digestion and health. Jaundice is a sign of liver dysfunction and in Chinese medicine we talk about Liver *Qi* stagnation, which in some patterns can lead to a build-up of dampness, which can cause jaundice. With some causes of stagnation we need to invigorate or circulate the blood, which both rosemary and exercise can do. Its use as a circulatory tonic makes it effective in not only helping with jaundice, but also with treating pain, digestive issues, varicose veins, poor memory, and depression.

Liver *Qi* stagnation can cause pain anywhere in the body. Rosemary has long been used for rheumatic pain. For many who have rheumatic pain, dampness is a factor in the chronic inflammation that leads to deformation of joints. The spicy nature of rosemary transforms dampness and releases toxicity from the body. Physical toxins like food poisoning or acidity in the blood, or emotional imbalances, such as the Seven Damages—worry, pensiveness, anger, grief, fear, fright, and mania—can lead to chronic pain, mental illness or disease. When emotions have affected our internal organs, as in the case of the Seven Damages, a person can have insomnia, nightmares, and even abnormal or incoherent thoughts and speech.

Liver *Qi* stagnation can also lead to a disturbance of the *Hun*. Our *Hun* is our ethereal soul, often described as three benevolent beings who aid you in the practice of compassionate action. Like a peaceful warrior, our *Hun* allows us to see past our obstacles and walk the righteous path. When our *Hun* gets disturbed, we may experience anger, frustration, indecision, or a lack of motivation or vision to accomplish our goals. Rosemary helps break up stagnation so the *Hun* can wander freely, moving between our liver and our eyes, giving insight and vision into the present and future.

Herb of Remembrance

A conserve made of rosemary can restore speech from something Gerard called "dumb palsy." The original meaning of dumb is "mute," and palsy is paralysis with tremors. It is unclear to me whether "dumb palsy" is a constitutional condition or can accompany a stroke or other neurological condition. Gerard also gives a recipe for sugar desserts from rosemary flowers to comfort the heart, to "make it merry, quicken the spirits and make them more lively." The association between rosemary and the heart, and as the symbolic herb for both love and death, dates back to antiquity.

Gerard, in his famous *Of the Historie of Plants*, speaks of *Rosmarinus coronaria*, called *coronaria* because women were known to make crowns and garlands from its branches. Maud Grieve, an early twentieth-century British herbalist who wrote extensively on plants, writes that the ancient Greeks viewed rosemary as the emblem of fidelity for lovers and as an emblem for remembrance in both weddings and funerals. A symbol of love and loyalty, a rosemary branch was tied with silken ribbons of all colors and presented to all wedding guests to ensure a marriage filled with enduring affection. The bride and groom wore rosemary to help them remember their love for each other throughout a lifetime of marriage.

Widely known as a wisdom herb in Western herbalism, rosemary brings deep insight into remembering who you really are. The Arabian physicians wrote that rosemary comforted the brain and the memory, drawing the senses inward. When the senses are drawn inward, we move into a deeper state of meditation where universal truths are more accessible. In these moments of clarity, we know who we are. We remember why we chose to be reborn. Through this clarity, we gain access to the wisdom and courage to do it all again.

Releasing Fear

Our modern lifestyle can greatly disturb our *Shen*. The continuous bombardment of war, natural disasters, political upheaval, and the constant use of electronic devices are rewiring our neural networks, creating postural changes, and replacing our personal, intimate relationships. This level of global information is new for the human species. It can be overwhelming for us psychologically as we struggle with a way to assimilate all the problems of the world. When our *Shen* is disturbed we can become fearful, agitated, restless, anxious and disconnected from the world around us. The technologically advanced, fast-paced lives many of us lead disrupt our endocrine and nervous systems and elicit a fight-or-flight reaction. This sympathetic nervous system response is natural, but becomes problematic when it occurs on a frequent basis. In fight-or-flight, the body temporarily shuts down its digestive and mental faculties and elicits a primal response of either fight/die or run/hide. Multiple episodes of shock, fright, and fear can deplete our kidney energy and affect our *Zhi*, the energy of willpower and will to live. I know that I have lived in a sympathetic state for much of my life. By the time I was nine years old I had been through countless procedures to find out why I had recurrent urinary tract infections. I was finally diagnosed with ureter reflux and had corrective surgery in the summer of 1985. We had to wait for school to be out for the summer, because I had to stay in the hospital for two weeks and then recover at home for another few weeks before I could resume normal activity. The months leading up to the surgery were torture. Not only did I still experience constant pain, but also now my mind went to dark places, like what if I died in surgery? My parents acted strong and convincing, but I saw and heard the doctor explain things to my mom on our numerous visits. It was a serious surgery and without it I could lose the function of not one, but both of my kidneys.

When I was six years old my older sister Lia was diagnosed with juvenile (type-1) diabetes. My parents began to notice that she was losing weight, although she was eating well. As her overall vitality decreased, she also began to have urinary incontinence at night. When the doctor saw her blood work, she was immediately admitted to Saint Jude Children's Hospital, which was near our home in Memphis. Lia and my mom spent a week in the hospital as Lia's blood sugar dropped and the ketones in her urine fell to safe levels. From the first time I heard about what diabetes is and what ketoacidosis means, I developed a fear of illness and death. It also clued me into the importance of our kidneys for our existence.

The diagnosis of my sister's illness shifted my awareness of life, death, and health. As I watched her struggle with the acceptance of a life-long condition, blood tests, insulin shots, and timed eating, the fear of her going into a diabetic coma began to infiltrate my daily thoughts. I think everyone in my family was afraid. My parents are strong, loving people, and they tried to assure me that Lia was going to be okay. I was encouraged to watch after her and make sure she checked her blood and took her shots. With the added responsibility of her health, I continued to be afraid for her. It wasn't until my urinary tract problems became daily instead of every few months that I began to fear for my own mortality as well.

Master Healer

My work with plant medicine has led me to rosemary to heal these deep wounds of identity and mortality. When my sister was diagnosed, part of my identity became one of caregiver. But by the time I had my surgery three years later, I could only think about my own mortality, as I spent months fighting infection and pain. I needed all my energy to heal.

These two traumatic childhood health conditions have followed me throughout my life. I have a tendency to imagine the worst-case scenario and instinctively I come from a place of fear. These are the reasons I was drawn to herbal and traditional medicine. They contributed to why I am an herbalist, acupuncturist, healer. In my life, I have witnessed that allopathic medicine is essential for emergency situations. I know that pharmaceutical intervention is the only way to save lives sometimes. I also know that our medical system is motivated by profit, and not necessarily health. It lacks greatly in addressing the psycho-spiritual-emotional approach to our bodies, which is essential to deep healing.

Rosemary was once widely used to rid a person of evil spirits and bad dreams. According to *Magical Herbalism: The Secret Craft of the Wise*, by Scott Cunningham, rosemary can prevent nightmares when placed under the pillow. I believe rosemary broke up the patterns of fear that have been ingrained in me since childhood. I have had countless cups of rosemary tea and invigorating baths with fresh rosemary twigs, but it is my work with rosemary essential oil where I have recalled who I was before these events occurred.

I often wear essential oils, applied as a roll-on in carrier oil. A couple of years ago I began to be attracted to wearing rosemary verbenone essential oil. It's not an intoxicating aroma, like those I usually prefer (amber, jasmine, vetiver), but it seemed necessary at the time. I felt like rosemary was calling me, enticing me to listen to what medicines lay inside. I placed a single drop on top of my head and waited. Within moments I saw images of myself as a small child, laughing, spinning, feeling completely innocent and free. There was a lightness beaming in all directions. Then there were visions of my sister's illness, my own infections and pain, and I felt the lightness turn to heaviness. My shoulders and chest tightened and contracted, and fear and sadness crept into my soul. At that moment rosemary said, *Remember, remember who you are.*

I cried large, sobbing tears for the little girl who did not know what it meant to live, or to die—only what it meant to be joyous and free of life's burdens. Once I released my attachment to what I had lost, I felt renewed. I was energized, clear, and happy. I knew that I didn't have to hold on to the fear as part of my identity, as part of my story. I remembered who I was before the trauma happened and I could tap into that energy to sustain and nourish myself.

Rosemary's Song

Rosemary is here to remind you of who you were before you lost your innocence. You will be vibrant, joyful and healthy when you remember who you are. Rosemary is your guide to becoming your authentic self.

Remember who you are
Be who you are meant to be

Rosemary Recipes

Rosemary Liniment

Fill a quart jar 1/3 full of fresh or dried rosemary sprigs. Pour witch hazel or alcohol over the sprigs, filling jar to 1" from the top. Cover jar and let sit for 4 weeks. Shake jar daily. After 1 month, strain out rosemary and save liquid in a glass jar. Label "for external use only." Use topically on sore muscles, strains and sprains.

Wisdom Tea

- 1 tbsp. Rosemary sprigs
- 8 ounces water

Bring water to a boil, add rosemary and decoct for 15 minutes. Strain out rosemary and drink decoction slowly as you meditate on your higher purpose in this life. Allow all thoughts to come without judgment or fear.

Awaken & Evoke Spray

- 3 drops rosemary essential oil
- 3 drops clary sage essential oil
- 3 drops tulsi basil essential oil
- 1 drop *Angelica archangelica* essential oil

Add essential oils to 1 ounce spring water. Pour into a glass spritzer bottle and shake well. Mist yourself as needed for inspiration, motivation or clarity.

Herbal Vinegar

- 3 sprigs of rosemary
- 4 ounces of apple cider vinegar or white wine vinegar

Place the rosemary sprigs in organic apple cider or wine vinegar and let steep for 1-2 weeks. Strain herbs if desired. The sour flavor of the vinegar, along with the medicinal properties of rosemary, make this one of the best ways to strengthen digestion. For flavoring, add 1-2 teaspoons on salads or cooked vegetables. For a medicinal dose, take 15 ml/per 100 pounds before meals.

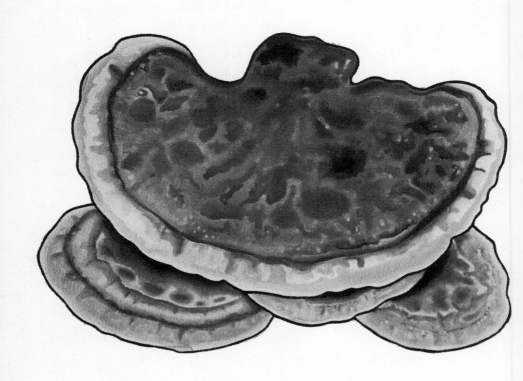

CHAPTER SIXTEEN

Reishi: Go Deep, Live Long

Ganoderma Lucidum
Reishi
Ling Zhi

- **Properties:** Sweet, Neutral
- **Meridians entered**: Heart, Liver, Kidney, Spleen, Lung
- **Elements influenced**: Fire, Wood, Water, Earth, Metal
- **Original habitat**: Temperate and subtropical North & South America, Europe, Asia.
- **Habitats**: On deciduous hardwood trees; cultivated on logs or wood chips.

Description: Reishi are hard, shiny, fan-shaped polypore mushrooms that grow on deciduous hardwood trees. The growing edge is cream colored and turns to darker shades of reddish brown as they age.

Go deep
Live long

Jessica Baker, LAc, RH (AHG)

Spirit Medicine

As our fascination with the properties of mycelium and mushrooms increases, so does our exploration of our evolutionary history with these celestial beings. Many theories and legends expound upon the mythical, magical properties of fungi. In Daoism, _Ling Zhi_ (spirit fungus) are said to belong to the Immortals, a group of highly advanced beings who can live outside our space and time and move between dimensions. One genus of fungus, _Ganoderma_, is said to be found only in the mountains where the Immortals dwell.

The _Shen Nong Ben Cao Jing_, or _The Divine Farmer's Materia Medica_, one of the oldest Chinese herbal texts, was compiled around 200 AD and first printed in 1803. Book One divides herbs into three categories: superior, medium, and inferior. The highest category is the superior medicines, said to nourish life and correspond to the heavens. Superior herbs are known to prevent illness, increase longevity, connect with the spirit world, and elevate the spiritual mind. Medium herbs nurture personality and correspond to humanity. Medium herbs are used to strengthen deficiencies, regulate _Qi_, or nourish yin. Herbs in this category may or may not be toxic. Inferior herbs treat disease and correspond to earth. These herbs strongly break up _Qi_ and blood stagnation and drive out heat or cold. Inferior herbs are toxic and cannot be taken for a long period of time. Guidance and knowledge of herbal formulation are necessary when using inferior herbs.

In the _Shen Nong Ben Cao Jing_, six different types of reishi mushrooms are noted as superior herbs, each variety named after its color. As noted in the chart in the opening pages, the color of an herb can correspond to emotions, parts of the body, and much more. With mushrooms, these color qualities have been well understood since the first or second century, if not earlier.

The spiritual connection between humans and mushrooms had long been established by the herbalists of that time. _Ling Zhi_ was known to prevent senility and prolong life so as to make one an Immortal—the only herb to receive such a distinction in the _Shen Nong_. There are several others that are said to boost _Qi_, or to make the body "light," which I interpret as a brightening of one's inner light. There are other herbs and fungi that are said to prolong life but it is only reishi that confers immortality. The Daoist monks understood time, space and our relationship to them in a much different way than we understand them today. Working with the spirit mushrooms, we, too, can enter the void, where space and time are no longer linear and do not adhere to our limitations and beliefs.

144

Modern Medicine

In modern Chinese medicine, *Ling Zhi* is still revered as an important *Qi* tonic, and much research has been done on this mystical fungi. One of the most bitter medicines known, polypore mushrooms have been researched in depth and are found to be one of the strongest immune-modulating substances in nature. *Ganoderma lucidum* has been shown to reduce tumor growth and increase immune response and white blood cell counts. As an antibiotic, *Ling Zhi* can lower and inhibit the growth of *E. coli*, dysentery, pseudomonas, pneumococci, streptococci, staphylococci and others. The research on the medicinal properties of these and other mushrooms are showing great potential for disease prevention.

Chinese Herbalism

The nature of *Ling Zhi* is sweet and neutral and has an affinity for the heart, liver, and lung. *Ling Zhi* nourishes the heart and calms the *Shen*. In Chinese medicine we know there is an intimate connection between the heart, the mind and the spirit. If one of the three are injured or disturbed, then all will be affected. With our fast-paced lifestyles and the constant bombardment of news of trauma from across the globe, our spirits are definitely being affected. I feel it within myself and I hear about it from my family, friends and clients.

My experience with *Ling Zhi* has been profound. I have had the most insightful meditations with just a few sips of an infusion. I love to make a solar-lunar infusion, sitting it outside for twenty-four hours, and then spending the next few days refilling the jar as I drink it down. I observe how the mushroom begins to make me feel. Immediately I notice that my heart rate decreases, the tension in my jaw relaxes, and my breath deepens. The difference is palpable and it always makes me smile. After the initial reactions, I experience a dense calmness, like time has slowed down and I can see everything a little more clearly. I am less reactive, more centered and subdued. I feel wonderfully expansive like I do in yoga, *Qi Gong* or meditation. It's similar to the way I feel in an old-growth redwood forest: alive, breathing at one with the planet. Profound truths become easier to hear, absorb, and transmute.

Mushroom Revolution

Someone who really hears the call of the mushrooms is Paul Stamets. He and his team have revolutionized the use of polypores for bio-remediation and hazardous and chemical-waste cleanup. They have open patents on several polypore technologies, including one using reishi mycelium extract in bee hives to prevent the spread of colony death and other hive diseases. We all know bees are essential for pollination, but most of us don't fully comprehend what that means for humanity. Bees are our main insect pollinators, contributing to many of the fruits and vegetables we eat today, along with fiber and livestock plants. Transporting bees across the United States during various pollination seasons is essential for large-scale agriculture as we know it. The California almond market, for example, would be ruined without this system.

As bee populations decline due to hive diseases, pesticide use, and a decrease of wild spaces, we become more aware of how integral they are to our lives. The winter of 2015-2016 was the worst year for colony death, with 44% of hives perishing. In 2014, Stamets teamed up with Washington State University to investigate whether or not exposing bees to mushroom extracts would reduce viral burden. Preliminary research is proving positive. At the time of this writing, the largest field study on bees to date is occurring, in which researchers administered extracts of *Ganoderma lucidum* and *Fomes fomentarius* (a fungus that grows on the sides of trees) to 532 bee hives in an attempt to strengthen the bees' immunity and prevent colony death.

Like the mycelium that allows fungus to communicate with the rest of the plant kingdom, we are intricately connected to all living beings. The decline of the bees is just another sign of our continued destruction. It is a wake-up call as to how human "progress" is affecting the rest of the planet.

Through rigorous research and sacred plant meditation we continue to explore the sensorial relationships we have with bees, mushrooms, and other forms of life. As genome mapping proves the fundamental truth that we are all one, that we are all related, that we are all part of this delicate thing called Life, humanity will once again remember our place in the balance of the Universe. We will quell our destructive natures and go deep inside again for the answers to the mysteries we seek to know.

Reishi's Song

We are Cosmic dust, we are of this Earth, and we are forged by the elements of nature. The Earth was here billions of years before humans emerged and she will continue to thrive long after we are gone. Humans are not necessary for the survival of the planet, but we do belong here. Our sensory communication with other beings, like mycelium, reminds us of our intrinsic connection to this planet.

Go deep
Live long

Jessica Baker, LAc, RH (AHG)

Reishi Recipes

Mushroom Moon Tea

Take 1-3 reishi mushrooms and place in one quart boiled water. Place in the moonlight (full moon is strongest). In the morning strain out mushrooms. Drink 1/2 cup tea before meditating. Allow the spirit mushroom to nourish your body and soul.

Reishi Rising

Place a 2-inch or larger reishi mushroom in 8 ounces of room-temperature water. Allow mushroom to infuse in the water for 3 days and 3 nights. Take out mushroom, making sure to strain out all mushroom debris. Add 1/8 ounce of brandy or vegetable glycerin to the water. Store in a glass bottle. Take 1-7 drops of the mushroom elixir as needed for clarity of thought.

Adaptogen Blend

1 ounce, powdered, of each of the following:

- reishi mushroom
- tulsi basil
- astragalus
- Siberian ginseng

Mix powdered herbs together. Fill "00" capsules with mixture. Take 1-2 capsules daily to increase energy and strengthen the body and soul.

CONCLUSION

These sixteen plants have shaped my life in ways I didn't even realize until I began this book. As I wrote, memories and sensations woke up parts of me that I had forgotten about. As rewarding as finishing a book is, it was also very hard for me to write out intimate details about my life. Some I only admit to myself as I read it coming out. Old wounds resurfaced and some found resolution. Others are raw again or just-realized, and I already hear the whispering of the plants, leading me towards the ones who will help me work through these as well.

Writing *Plant Songs* reminded me of the evolutionary miracles of life on Earth, long before humans existed. I remembered humanity's reliance on plants for food, medicine, fiber, and shelter. I recalled how humans and plants breathe together, live together, and evolve together. I thought about our disconnection from nature, from the plants, from each other. I know that so much of our physical, emotional, and spiritual pain is because we lost our kinship with plants. We have forgotten that we are part of the ecosystem; we forgot we are part of this Earth.

I hope that by reading *Plant Songs* you are encouraged to spend more time in nature, or to listen to your rosemary bush, or to hug the nearest tree. My desire is that you find peace in knowing that nature provides solutions to your pain, your grief, or your discontent. I urge you to rekindle your relationships with the plants whom call to you. Listen to them, and believe what you hear.

My hope for you is that you become an advocate for the Earth, for others, and most of all, for yourself. To begin, just sit back, listen closely, and listen to the songs of the plants.

ACKNOWLEDGEMENTS

I thank my soulmate and husband Chip Baker for his encouragement and support in my passion for herbalism and Chinese medicine. It is because of him that I believe I am capable of achieving anything I put my heart and mind towards. Fueled by his love, I have reached for the stars and put down my deepest roots.

I have the deepest gratitude to my parents for the sacrifices they made to raise two daughters in a loving, stable environment despite our transitory upbringing. My dad, Wayne Harrell, instilled in me a love of science fiction, gardening, and hiking in nature, all things that have led me to plant medicine. My mom, Sondra Koch, gifted me her resiliency and love of travel, two attributes that truly define who I am. I thank my sister, Lia Harrell, for being my first teacher, best friend and confidant. I am grateful for our lifelong friendship.

I have had many teachers over the years, but I would like to personally thank my herb teachers. It is because of them that I have remembered my intimate connection with plants. Thank you Jane Bothwell, Dr. Christopher Hobbs, PhD, Rosemary Gladstar, Julie Caldwell, Sharon Feng, and Jeffrey Yuen for sharing your love of herbalism. I also thank all of my clients for their willingness to heal their deepest wounds. Their courage allows me to do the same.

Thank you to Hay House for the Writer's Workshop. Winning a Balboa Press contract gave me the confidence to complete this book. Much gratitude to kn literary and my editor, Jason Buchholz. Jason's encouragement and kind words made writing this book less daunting and intimidating.

Finally, I am most grateful for the plants and fungi for sharing their songs with me. Their wisdom runs deep.